CONSCIOUS SEDATION

CONSCIOUS SEDATION

Jeanine P. Wiener-Kronish, M.D.

Professor and Vice-Chair
Department of Anesthesia
University of California San Francisco
San Francisco, California

Michael A. Gropper, M.D., Ph.D.

Associate Professor
Department of Anesthesia
Director, Critical Care Medicine
University of California San Francisco
San Francisco, California

HANLEY & BELFUS, INC. / Philadelphia

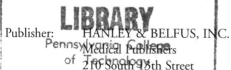
Publisher: HANLEY & BELFUS, INC.
Medical Publishers
210 South 13th Street
Philadelphia, PA 19107
(215) 546-7293; 800-962-1892
FAX (215) 790-9330
Web site: http://www.hanleyandbelfus.com

Note to the reader: Although the information in this book has been carefully reviewed for correctness of dosage and indications, neither the authors nor the editors nor the publisher can accept any legal responsibility for any errors or omissions that may be made. Neither the publisher nor the editors make any warranty, expressed or implied, with respect to the material contained herein. Before prescribing any drug, the reader must review the manufacturer's current product information (package inserts) for accepted indications, absolute dosage recommendations, and other information pertinent to the safe and effective use of the product described.

Library of Congress Cataloging-in-Publication Data

Conscious Sedation / edited by Jeanine P. Wiener-Kronish, Michael A. Gropper.
    p.   cm.
  Includes bibliographical references and index.
  ISBN 1-56053-413-3 (alk. paper)
  1. Conscious sedation. 2. Intravenous anesthesia.
  I. Wiener-Kronish, Jeanine P., 1951– . II. Gropper, Michael A., 1958– .
  [DNLM: 1. Conscious Sedation. WO 200 C755 2001]
  RD85.C64 C66 2001
  617.9'6—dc21

                                  00-063365

CONSCIOUS SEDATION   ISBN 1-56053-413-3

Last digit is the print number: 9 8 7 6 5 4 3 2 1

CONTENTS

CONTRIBUTORS

Edwin S. Cheng, M.D.
Resident, Department of Anesthesia, University of California San Francisco School of Medicine, San Francisco, California

Michael A. Gropper, M.D., Ph.D.
Associate Professor, Department of Anesthesia, Director, Critical Care Medicine, University of California San Francisco School of Medicine, San Francisco, California

Andrew Infosino, M.D.
Assistant Professor of Anesthesiology and Pediatrics, University of California San Francisco School of Medicine, San Francisco, California

Richard J. Kelly, M.D., J.D., M.P.H.
Anesthesiologist, San Francisco, California

Miranda Kramer, M.S., R.N., N.P., CCRN
Clinical Nurse and Nurse Practitioner, Department of Surgery, University of California San Francisco School of Medicine, San Francisco, California

Susan C. Lambe, M.D.
Robert Wood Johnson Clinical Scholar, Department of General Internal Medicine, UCLA School of Medicine, Los Angeles, California

Ludwig H. Lin, M.D.
Assistant Clinical Professor, Department of Anesthesia, University of California San Francisco School of Medicine, San Francisco, California

Linda L. Liu, M.D.
Assistant Clinical Professor, Department of Anesthesia, University of California San Francisco School of Medicine, San Francisco, California

Stephen B. Mooney, M.D.
Clinical Fellow, Division of Reproductive Endocrinology and Infertility, Department of Gynecology and Obstetrics, Stanford University School of Medicine, Stanford, California

Claus Niemann, M.D.

Clinical Instructor, Department of Anesthesia, University of California San Francisco School of Medicine, San Francisco, California

Susan M. Ryan, Ph.D., M.D.

Assistant Clinical Professor, Division of Critical Care, Department of Anesthesia, University of California San Francisco School of Medicine, San Francisco, California

Richard H. Savel, M.D.

Postdoctoral Fellow, Department of Anesthesia, University of California San Francisco School of Medicine, San Francisco, California

Lynn M. Westphal, M.D.

Assistant Professor, Division of Reproductive Endocrinology and Infertility, Department of Gynecology and Obstetrics, Stanford University School of Medicine, Stanford, California

Jeanine P. Wiener-Kronish, M.D.

Professor and Vice-Chair, Department of Anesthesia, University of California San Francisco School of Medicine, San Francisco, California

C. Spencer Yost, M.D.

Associate Professor, Department of Anesthesia, University of California San Francisco School of Medicine, San Francisco, California

PREFACE

Patients increasingly undergo procedures that require conscious sedation in both inpatient and outpatient settings. Conscious sedation is administered by medical personnel who may or may not have had formal education regarding such sedation. This has led to complications and even deaths in outpatient settings, particularly in cosmetic surgery cases—hence the need for this handbook. It was written to help practitioners provide safe conscious sedation that also results in patient satisfaction. Every practitioner involved in the administration of sedation or parenteral analgesia should be aware of the topics covered in this book.

A preprocedural evaluation always must be done and the criteria for exclusion or denial of conscious sedation are covered in the chapter on patient evaluation. The practitioners administering conscious sedation should be aware of the physical requirements and equipment that must be present to meet the Joint Commission on Accreditation of Healthcare Organizations (JCAHO) standards and to ensure patient safety; these issues are covered in the chapter on sedation in the outpatient setting. The chapters on pharmacology and reversal of conscious sedation cover the classification and pharmacology of agents used in conscious sedation and their antidotes.

The chapters regarding specific situations or patients are meant to be useful for practitioners caring for certain patient populations (elderly, pediatric, or critically ill patients) or providing specific procedures (endoscopy, emergency department, or assisted reproductive procedures). There is also a chapter for nurses, as their concerns and responsibilities are somewhat different from those of physicians. Finally, there is a chapter on the medical-legal issues regarding conscious sedation, which are important for all practitioners who engage in this activity.

We have tried to cover the major medical issues related to conscious sedation in a complete yet practical volume. We hope this text will be useful to physicians, nurses, and students in any specialty and setting involving conscious sedation.

Jeanine P. Wiener-Kronish, M.D.
Michael A. Gropper, M.D., Ph.D.

DEDICATION

The editors wish to dedicate this book to their spouses, Daniel
Kronish, MD, and Lynn Westphal, MD, as the time required
for this project was available only because of their generosity.
The editors also want to thank the contributing authors for
their thoughtful and careful work.

1

Pharmacology of Conscious Sedation

Claus Niemann, M.D.
Michael A. Gropper, M.D., Ph.D.

Conscious sedation is aimed for a patient population undergoing diagnostic or minor surgical procedures. This may include diagnostic magnetic resonance imaging (MRI), dental procedures, creation of arteriovenous (AV) fistulas, cataract surgery, upper/lower gastrointestinal flexible endoscopy, and many more. The requirements of a procedure may dictate that a certain population be sedated. For example, the lack of movement required for performing MRI scanning is often impossible for the youngest and oldest patients. Likewise, patients scheduled for eye surgery or AV fistulas often have coexisiting medical conditions that need to be carefully considered in the preoperative evaluation.

Furthermore, an increased number of procedures requiring conscious sedation are performed outside the operating room and sedation and analgesia are not always administered by an anesthesiologist. In order to develop an individualized plan for conscious sedation, the provider needs to consider the entire medical history (including medication) of the patient and define clinical endpoints, which allows him/her to guide pharmacologic intervention. A patient requiring conscious sedation should be able to respond appropriately to commands and be able to maintain a patent airway independently at all times. Yet, the patient wants to be comfortable and the physician performing the procedure desires cooperation and optimal operating conditions. The desired clinical endpoint of conscious sedation is, therefore, rather dynamic and not always achieved. Patient variability, the patient's medical problems, and the procedure (level of surgical stimulus) can have profound impact on the individual response to the administered drugs and might result in unsatisfactory conditions, including agitation, loss of consciousness, and lack of ventilation and hypoxemia.

While patient characteristics and the procedure cannot be modified, the pharmacologic intervention can be adjusted in terms of the drugs chosen and the doses administered. These choices require an understanding of pharmacologic principles, their application in clinical situations, and knowledge of the

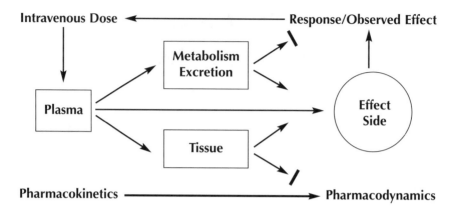

Figure 1. Dose-response relationship for a drug described by pharmacokinetics and pharmacodynamics. (Modified from Collins VJ (ed): Physiologic and Pharmacologic Bases of Anesthesia. Baltimore, Williams & Wilkins, 1996, with permission.)

factors that alter a patient's response to a given drug and dosing requirements. In general, the selection of a given drug should be based on a specific therapeutic goal and the pharmacologic properties and effect of the drug. For example, a patient who becomes increasingly agitated secondary to pain should be given a small dose of an opiate, rather than another sedative. Consequently, reaching a desired clinical endpoint requires vigilance, continuous assessment of the clinical situation, and knowledge of the drugs administered. This chapter reviews basic pharmacologic principles with a focus on their application in the setting of conscious sedation. Furthermore, the drugs commonly used for conscious sedation are discussed and reviewed. It is hoped that this chapter will provide the basis for delivery of conscious sedation by health care professionals in a safe and well-informed manner.

Basic Pharmacologic Principles

The decision to medicate a patient is not only influenced by a desired clinical endpoint, but also by the duration required for the drug-induced effect. Patients with chronic conditions such as hypertension require lifelong treatment. The time to onset, duration, variability, and intensity of response to a drug is measured in days and weeks. Therefore, oral administration of antihypertensive drugs, despite unpredictable absorption and an initially fluctuating plasma concentration, is acceptable for chronic treatment. However, the opposite is true for patients who require conscious sedation. The time frame of treatment is measured in minutes to a few hours. Clearly, this makes oral administration of drugs

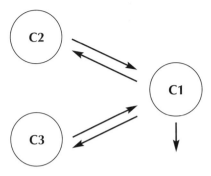

Figure 2. A three-compartment model with intercompartmental clearances and elimination clearance.

unacceptable, except for some pediatric procedures. The intravenous administration of drugs avoids the delay caused by absorption. Consequently, the intravenous administration of drugs is preferable for conscious sedation, as a given response to the drug administration is more predictable. A dose-response relationship of a drug, regardless of the route of administration, is defined by its pharmacokinetics and pharmacodynamics. This relationship is depicted in Figure 1.

Pharmacokinetics

It is well established that the magnitude of any given drug effect is a function of the concentration of the drug surrounding the site of action. Since the concentration at the action site cannot be measured in most cases, the plasma concentration of a drug is used as an approximation. The objective of any pharmacologic treatment is to maintain a therapeutic drug concentration at the site of action, hence optimal drug therapy requires knowledge of processes and mechanisms that can modify plasma drug concentrations. Compartmental and physiologic models are used in an attempt to predict plasma concentrations in the body after drug administration. The drugs used for conscious sedation can be described by a two- or three-compartment model. The modeling approach allows the determination of the relationship between a given drug dose, the time since administration, and the measured plasma concentration.

The physiologic effect is also considered in pharmacologic models. These models are used to explain the interaction between a drug and its receptor. It is essential to understand the basics of pharmacokinetic modeling, since all clinically employed pharmacokinetic parameters are model-based and using the wrong model obviously could result in devastating consequences for the patient. Figure 2 illustrates a simple three-compartment model with intercompartmental clearances and elimination clearance.

Pharmacokinetics models processes in the body and describes their impact on an administered drug. These processes, which determine the time course of drug action, can be subdivided into drug absorption, distribution, and elimination. While most drugs for conscious sedation are administered intravenously, it is important to understand certain principles of absorption. Bioavailability of a drug is defined as the fraction (in percentage) of the administered dose of a drug that reaches the systemic circulation. Absorption of drugs injected intramuscularly is often faster than oral administration; however, factors such as blood flow to the site of injection and infection at the site of injection can influence absorption of a drug and subsequently alter the drug concentration at the site of action. Intravenous injection offers instantaneous and complete absorption. Once the drug reaches the systemic circulation, it will be distributed to various tissues depending on factors such as regional blood flow, organ size, and the physicochemical properties of the drug.

Distribution describes the mixing and ongoing equilibration among the tissues. Distribution is most important early, during the rapid decline in the plasma drug concentration immediately following an intravenous bolus dose. During this time, very little of the drug has been eliminated; there may be a decline in the pharmacologic effect of some drugs in this distribution phase. Some drugs distribute faster to their site of action than to the peripheral tissues; this pattern is associated with a rapid onset of action. The redistribution of the drug to slower-equilibrating tissues will shorten the duration of the pharmacologic effect when a single intravenous dose is given. The onset and offset of many drugs used in anesthesia and conscious sedation are distribution-dependent and follow this rule. A commonly used term to describe the distribution of drugs is *volume of distribution* (Vd). It can be described as the volume in which a drug appears to be homogeneously distributed in the body. Vd can be defined as the volume of plasma at a given drug concentration required to account for all the amount of drug in the body. The following equation depicts this relationship:

$$Vd = A/C$$

where A is the amount of drug in the body and C the plasma drug concentration.

While the volume of distribution gives information about the distribution of an injected drug, certain requirements are necessary for the accurate determination of Vd. The amount of drug in the body needs to be known and an equilibrium between the plasma and the tissues has to be achieved. Furthermore, the drug has to partition to all tissues equally in order for the apparent volume of distribution to be an accurate estimate of the actual tissue volume. It becomes obvious that calculating Vd during the early distribution phase would result in erroneous estimates for the Vd, since the plasma concentration is not in equilibrium with the tissues. In addition, there is no physical space equal to the Vd.

Drugs strongly bound to tissues may have very low plasma concentrations even though the total amount of the drug in the body is high. Therefore, the Vd may be significantly greater than the total volume of the body.

Conversely, a drug that is not highly bound to tissues, but remains in the plasma, will have a Vd that approximates the plasma volume. Consequently, the Vd can be modified by alterations in plasma binding (e.g., liver disease), blood vessel permeability, and other factors.

Elimination clearance (CL_E) is a pharmacokinetic parameter that describes various processes that decrease the amount of drug in the body. As volume of distribution relates concentration to the amount of drug, elimination clearance is used to relate concentration to the rate of drug elimination and can be mathematically described as follows:

$$Clearance = k \times Vd$$

where k is a first-order constant characterizing the elimination process and is therefore known as elimination rate constant. The elimination rate constant can be described as:

$$k = \text{rate of elimination/amount in body} \rightarrow (CL_E \times C) / (Vd \times C) \rightarrow CL_E/Vd$$

$$k = CL_E/Vd$$

Most drugs follow first-order kinetics in that the rate of drug elimination is directly proportional to the drug concentration in the plasma.

Elimination clearance is the parameter that characterizes the removal of a drug from the body. It can be defined as the part of the volume of distribution from which a drug is irreversibly removed per unit of time and therefore relates to the termination of drug effect. Clearance elimination is the sum of individual organ clearances of a particular drug such as renal, hepatic, and pulmonary clearances.

Organ clearances, in turn, depend on factors such as organ blood flow, extraction of a drug by a given organ, and conditions and disease states that decrease organ function. Although renal elimination can be approximated by the creatinine clearance, hepatic clearance of drugs cannot be predicted accurately from standard liver tests. Genetic factors, hepatic blood flow, and metabolic activity (P-450 cytochrome) are some of the factors that determine hepatic clearance. Genetic deficiencies, altered hepatic blood flow, or decreased enzyme activity from disease can profoundly modify hepatic clearance of drugs and therefore make estimations of hepatic clearance unpredictable.

In contrast to elimination clearance, elimination half-life is a descriptive term used to characterize the relationship between the plasma concentration of a drug over time. It is not a primary pharmacokinetic parameter since it is completely determined by the volume of distribution and by clearance. The concept of the half-life of a drug is the time for the amount or concentration of an administered drug to fall to one-half its value at some previous time. Elimination half-life can be derived mathematically and described as follows:

$$T_{1/2} = 0.693 \times k \rightarrow T_{1/2} = 0.693 \, CL_E/Vd$$

where 0.693 represents the natural log of 2 (which is mathematically derived) and k is a first-order rate constant that, as we have seen above, is entirely defined by CL_E and Vd. Elimination half-life is of minor importance for drugs used for conscious sedation; as most of the drugs used in this setting are administered as a single bolus, the offset of drug effect is due to the drug's redistribution from the site of action. However, elimination half-life is important when selecting intervals for drug dosing, predicting drug accumulation, preventing adverse drug reactions, and determining the time necessary to achieve a steady-state drug concentration. Intra- and inter-individual variability of elimination half-lives are caused by extremes of age, sex, weight, and diseases. In fact, these clinical factors are reflected in changes in Vd and CL_E. Health care professionals need to assess clearances of drugs and often come to the conclusion that elimination half-life is prolonged due to decreased CL_E. While it can happen, in many cases it is not the elimination half-life that changes, but rather the Vd decreases.

Pharmacodynamics

Once the drug has entered the systemic circulation, it is distributed throughout the body and metabolized, and if enough drug reaches the site of action, there is a physiologic change. Pharmacodynamics can be defined as the quantitative analysis of the relationship between the drug concentration at the site of action and the magnitude of the induced effect. However, in order to have an effect on the target cell, a signal has to be transduced through the cell membrane. Most of the drugs appear to work on protein structures such as receptors, ion channels, or ion pumps; these interactions lead to the production of second messengers that complete the communication between the extra- and intracellular spaces. The affinity of a drug to a receptor is one determining factor dictating the concentration of drug necessary to elicit a response. The affinity defines the potency of a drug and it is important to notice that this is a concentration-responsive relationship. If it were a dose-responsive relationship, pharmacokinetic factors would greatly influence the relationship and make determination of the potency of a drug difficult. In contrast to potency, drug efficacy describes the maximum effect any given drug can produce and is a surrogate for the intrinsic activity of the drug and its interaction with a receptor.

The factors that are important in producing a pharmacologic effect include the affinity and the interaction of drugs with a particular receptor and a requirement for a critical amount of drug interacting with the receptors. To obtain an effect from some drugs requires a large quantity of drug on the receptors; these drugs have very small differences between their therapeutic concentrations and their toxic concentrations. The steepness of the slope of the dose-response relationship illustrates this relationship and provides information on how to titrate a drug to obtain an effect. A steep slope indicates that a small increase in the dose can produce a large increase in the pharmacologic effect.

Drug Interactions

Drug interactions in the treatment of patients with multiple medical problems are commonly observed. Knowledge and anticipation on part of the health care provider can avoid harming the patient. Drug interactions can be defined as follows: "A potential drug interaction refers to the possibility that one drug may alter the intensity of pharmacologic effects of another drug given concurrently. The net result maybe enhanced or diminished effects of one or both drugs or the appearance of a new effect that is not seen with either drug alone" (Goodman and Gilman).[4]

However, the absence of clinical evidence of a drug–drug interaction should not be misinterpreted as the lack of interaction. Manifestations of drug–drug interactions in a particular setting may be too subtle to be clinically detected. In fact, the same drug combination might cause serious harm to the patient in a different setting or when given in different dosages.

Serious side effects and toxicity are often seen with drugs that have a low therapeutic index, where small changes in drug concentration can potentially have severe adverse outcomes. Subsequent analysis or systematic research often can elucidate whether a drug–drug interaction is related to pharmacokinetics or pharmacodynamics. Pharmacokinetic drug interactions can result from a variety of mechanisms, including altered bioavailability, drug distribution, and metabolism/clearance. Any drugs given concurrently can interfere with one of the above-stated factors and thus change the drug concentration of the other drug at the target site and therefore its profile. This kind of drug interaction is based on pharmacokinetic alterations.

The binding site of a receptor for a given drug is rather specific and is defined by factors such as the drug affinity. Drug–drug interaction can also take place at the target site without being influenced by pharmacokinetics. Once the drug has reached its target site, its effect might be altered by other drugs competing for the same receptor. This interaction, a form of antagonism (competitive, irreversible, physiologic) can alter the dose-response curve of the drug of interest and hence change its therapeutic profile.

Even when the mechanism of drug–drug interaction is not at the receptor site, pharmacodynamic interaction can be demonstrated. For example, halothane, a volatile anesthetic, increases the frequency of arrythymias, and this propensity is further exaggerated by any drug that enhances sympathetic tone. The information

TABLE 1. Pharmacologic Properties of Benzodiazepines

Benzodiazepine	Potency	Distribution Volume (l/kg)	Clearance (ml/kg/min)	Protein Binding	Lipid Solubility
Midazolam	2–3	0.7–1.7	0.2–0.5	++++	+++
Diazepam	1	0.8–1.3	0.8–1.8	++++	+++
Lorazepam	4–10	1–1.7	6.4–11	++++	+++

on whether a potential drug–drug interaction is due to interference in pharmacokinetics or in pharmacodynamics is important for drug selection.

Benzodiazepines

Benzodiazepines are commonly used for conscious sedation because they have desirable properties such as anxiolysis, sedation, antegrade amnesic action, and muscle relaxation. All compounds in this class have various degrees of lipophilicity and protein binding. The various drugs thus differ in their pharmacokinetics. For instance, while substances with high lipophilicity such as diazepam, flurazepam, and triazolam are rapidly and completely absorbed from the gastrointestinal tract, substances such as midazolam have a slower onset and are less completely absorbed from the gastrointestinal tract. The ideal route of administration for conscious sedation, as already discussed, appears to be intravenous. With the exception of a selected pediatric population and the very anxious patient who might need sedation the night prior to the procedure, all benzodiazepines should be administered intravenously.

The majority of benzodiazepines are metabolized by the liver by oxidation and conjugation. Diazepam and midazolam are metabolized through oxidation, and drugs known to interfere with the oxidative pathway, such as isoniazid, estrogens, and cimetidine can interfere with the liver degradation of benzodiazepines. Therefore, the level of drug for a given dose will be higher in these patients. Similarly, age and liver disease have been shown to be major factors influencing the oxidative metabolism of benzodiazepines; for instance, the elderly have 50% of the "normal" clearance of benzodiazepines. In addition, some substances, such as diazepam, have active metabolites (e.g., desmethyldiazepam) that can enhance/prolong the effects of the parent drug and therefore render the drug effect unpredictable. Obviously, this is a particular risk in the older patient population. Lorazepam is primarily metabolized via glucuronide conjugation and thus is less prone to be influenced by coadministered drugs or by coexisting liver disease.

The mechanism of action of benzodiazepines is thought to be through the gamma-aminobutyric acid (GABA) receptors in the brain. GABA causes central inhibition. Benzodiazepines modify the GABA-related sodium channels and enhance the inhibitory effects of GABA; for instance, benzodiazepines increase sedation. While the GABA-receptor complex is ubiquitous in the brain, the most important site of action for benzodiazepines appears to be in postsynaptic modification after GABA stimulation.

The desired effects of benzodiazepines are amnesia and sedation, which makes their use reasonable in procedures with minimal to no pain. However, it should be kept in mind that there is often a discrepancy between the extent of amnesia and the level of sedation. Profound amnesia might be present in the patient, yet his or her level of consciousness may be less affected. Obviously this would be entirely appropriate for a cooperative, calm patient undergoing MRI scanning, but unacceptable for a restless patient scheduled for the same procedure. The effect of benzodiazepines on different organ systems is minimal to moderate. Even at large doses, benzodiazepines have minimal effects on the cardiovascular system. Given as a single drug, benzodiazepines cause only minimal decline in blood pressure, systemic vascular resistance, and cardiac output; however, these changes are dose-related. In general, midazolam causes a slightly greater decrease in blood pressure that other benzodiazepines. Central respiratory depression and even apnea can occur with benzodiazepines and are dose-related.

Severe adverse affects of benzodiazepines occur when they are given with other drugs, such as opioids and barbiturates. Given in combination with these drugs, cardiovascular perturbations (e.g., decrease in blood pressure) are greater and hemodynamic consequences may become clinically significant. The depressive effect on spontaneous ventilation is markedly enhanced when narcotics are used in combination with benzodiazepines, and apnea can occur.

Midazolam is probably most commonly used for preoperative sedation and short procedures involving conscious sedation. Its popularity is mainly due to its rapid onset and relatively short duration, which is due to its rapid clearance from the blood. The time of maximal central nervous system effect is somewhat variable but is in general is considered to be less than 4 minutes. However, the dose-response curve of midazolam is steeper than for other benzodiazepines such as diazepam. This implies that small changes in dosage of midazolam can result in an exaggerated clinical response. If multiple doses of midazolam are administered over a short period of time, there can be an accumulation of the drug, which puts the patient at risk of experiencing adverse side effects, such as respiratory depression and apnea. Although diazepam and lorazepam are available as intravenous agents, their use has significantly decreased after the introduction of midazolam.

TABLE 2. Pharmacologic Properties of Opioids

Opioid	Potency	Distribution Volume (l/kg)	Clearance (ml/kg/min)	Protein Binding	Lipid Solubility
Morphine	1	3-5	15–30	+	+
Alfentanil	25	0.4–1.0	4–9	++++	++
Fentanyl	100	3–5	10–20	+++	+++
Meperidine	0.1	3–5	8–18	++	+

This is mainly secondary to their unfavorable pharmacokinetic and pharmacodynamic profile for conscious sedation procedures. Their onset of action is significantly longer than for midazolam and the duration of effect more prolonged. Lorazepam is particularly unpredictable with regard to duration and is not an ideal choice for procedures of short duration requiring early discharges.

Opioids

Opioids are an important component of conscious sedation for patients undergoing potentially painful procedures. Since hypnotic drugs, with the exception of ketamine, do not possess any analgesic properties, a combination of a benzodiazepine and an opioid is often administered to patients to ensure sedation and analgesia. Opioids have various degrees of lipophilicity and protein binding, with morphine having the lowest and fentanyl and sufentanil having the highest protein binding and lipid solubility. Again, as expected, the physicochemical properties of each substance are in part responsible for the pharmacokinetics of each drug. Morphine's low lipid solubility results in a slow onset and a prolonged duration. The rapid onset and shorter duration of fentanyl and sufentanil can be attributed to their high lipid solubility. Alfentanil, although less lipid-soluble, has an even faster onset and shorter duration than fentanyl, probably due to an increased nonionized fraction and smaller volume of distribution, which enhances the amount of drug available at the receptor site. After a single bolus or small repeated doses, redistribution is the main factor that terminates the action of opioids. The effects of larger doses or infusions will mainly depend on biotransformation.

With the exception of remifentanil, an opioid not recommended for conscious sedation (see below), all available opioids are biotransformed in the liver and their hepatic clearance is flow-dependent (high hepatic extraction ratio). Since elimination half-life is defined in part by volume of distribution, alfentanil with the smallest volume of distribution possesses the shortest elimination half-life of opioids cleared by the liver.

Of importance, there are active metabolites formed after the administration of morphine and meperidine. In fact, morphine-6-glucuronide is an active metabolite of morphine that is more potent and longer-lasting than its parent drug. Since the elimination of the metabolites depends on renal function, renal failure can lead to prolonged ventilatory depression and sedation. Similarly, normeperidine, an active metabolite of meperidine, can lead, in a dose-dependent fashion, to central nervous system excitation and seizures. As with morphine-6-glucoronide, normeperidine may accumulate in patients with renal failure and should be used with caution in this patient population.

The mechanism of action of opioids is mediated through opioid receptors, which are distributed throughout the central nervous system, including the spinal cord, peripheral nerves, and other organs such as the gastrointestinal tract. Different receptor types, such as mu, kappa, and sigma receptors, have been identified and the clinical effect of opioids depends in part on the type of receptor stimulated by the particular opioid. For instance, dysphoria is mediated by a different receptor than analgesia. Another effect of opioid administration is pruritus. While the underlying mechanism is not well understood (it can occur after the administration of intravenous or spinal opioids) the pattern of pruritus appears to be fairly consistent. The face, in particular the nose, seems to be prone to itching. Naloxone, an opioid antagonist, is able to reverse the effect, suggesting histamine release is not involved. Pupillary constriction is mediated by the inhibition of the Edinger-Westphal nucleus in the brain. Nausea and vomiting, triggered by stimulation of the medullary chemoreceptor zone, can pose a significant problem in certain patients treated with opioids. These symptoms and problems can be treated with droperidol or seretonin reuptake inhibitors.

The effect of opioids on the cardiovascular system depends on which opioid is administered. Meperidine is the only opioid that can elicit direct myocardial depression in clinically relevant doses. Furthermore, meperidine tends to increase the heart rate as opposed to other opioids such as fentanyl, which tend to reduce sympathetic tone and can induce vagus-mediated bradycardia, particularly with increasing doses. As a consequence, a decrease in blood pressure can often be observed after meperidine administration, especially when patients are not stimulated. This decrease in blood pressure can be exaggerated and become clinically relevant in patients receiving other drugs such as hypnotics or benzodiazepines. Meperidine and morphine also may cause histamine release, resulting in significant hypotension. Patients whose blood pressure is elevated by sympathetic tone (pain) will also experience hypotension with opiate administration. This is not a direct effect of the drug; rather, the relief of pain decreases sympathetic tone, resulting in hypotension.

Ventilatory depression is often associated with opioid administration and the extent of respiratory depression depends on the dose administered and other factors, including the general health of the patient. In general, respiratory rate is decreased while tidal volume is preserved or increased. Minute ventilation, despite adequate tidal volumes, is not maintained due to a disproportionate decrease in respiratory rate. Increased carbon dioxide levels can be observed. Furthermore, ventilatory response to increased carbon dioxide and decreased oxygen is blunted, placing the patient at additional risk for hypoventilation and hypoxemia. Histamine release after the administration of morphine or meperidine can induce bronchospam in susceptible patients. Chest wall rigidity, documented after the administration of large doses of fentanyl, sufentanil, remifentanil, and alfentanil, can be avoided by slower administration and smaller doses of these drugs. Opioids also tend to increase the resting tone of the gastrointestinal tract. As a result, gastric emptying is delayed and peristalsis is reduced. Furthermore, opioids can increase the muscle tone of the sphincter of Oddi. This may lead to spasm and biliary colic in susceptible patients and may interfere with cholangiography.

The most frequently used opioid by nonanesthesiologists is probably meperidine. The potency of meperidine is approximately one tenth of morphine's. Aside from the potential risk of accumulation of its metabolite, normeperidine, the combination of meperidine with monoamine oxidase inhibitors can result in a life-threatening condition associated with severe hypertension, respiratory arrest, elevated temperature, and coma. While this can occur with any opioid, meperidine seems to be associated with this syndrome more frequently. The mechanism of this drug interaction is not well understood. A feature unique to meperidine is its ability to attenuate or terminate shivering in patients. This effect is particularly observed in patients having received general or regional (e.g., epidural catheter) anesthesia. The mechanism of this reaction is not known.

Fentanyl and alfentanil are approximately 100 times and 25 times more potent than morphine, respectively. Consequently, both drugs are significantly more potent than meperidine. This is an important distinction and should be kept in mind when using these drugs. Naturally, the margin of safety with regard to side effects such as respiratory depression is decreased in comparison to meperidine. Fentanyl and alfentanil have rapid onsets of action and alfentanil is a good choice for very short procedures with moderate to intense pain, such as a retrobulbar block for eye surgery. However, as in every case, communication with the eye surgeon is essential since some surgeons prefer a hypnotic over opioids due to the increased incidence of nausea and vomiting after opioid administration.

Morphine, sufentanil, and remifentanil are probably not ideal opioids for conscious sedation. Morphine has a slow onset of action, which makes rapid titration difficult and its prolonged effect is undesirable, especially in procedures

TABLE 3. Pharmacologic Properties of Hypnotic Agents

Hypnotic Agent	Distribution Volume (l/kg)	Clearance (ml/kg/min)	Protein Binding	Lipid Solubility
Thiopental	2.3	3.4	+++	+++
Methohexital	2.2	10.9	+++	+++
Propofol	2.8	59	++++	++++
Ketamine	3.1	19	+	++++

with minimal to moderate postprocedural pain. Sufentanil is extremely potent (500–1000 times as potent as morphine) and should almost exclusively be used by anesthesiologists. Due to its rapid biotransformation, remifentanil needs to be administered as an infusion except for very short procedures. Given the established safe use of alfentanil in this setting, remifentanil, with its higher potency and atypical pharmacokinetic behavior, appears to be ill-suited for nonanesthesiologists.

Hypnotic Agents

Hypnotic agents used for conscious sedation belong to different drug classes and therefore are discussed separately. Barbiturates, mainly methohexital and occasionally thiopental, are used frequently for conscious sedation. In addition, propofol has gained increased acceptance due its favorable pharmacokinetic and pharmacodynamic properties. Ketamine is used under certain circumstances, such as when the patient is uncooperative; it is not widely used because of its psychomimetic properties.

Barbiturates

The most commonly used barbiturates for conscious sedation are methohexital and thiopental. This is mainly due to their rapid onset and short duration of action in comparison to other barbiturates. As for almost all drugs discussed, the rapid onset is due to their physicochemical properties and the termination of their effects by redistribution away from the site of action. However, when given to patients as a continuous infusion to maintain sedation, recovery is faster after methohexital than after thiopental. Both drugs are metabolized in the liver but the hepatic extraction ratio for thiopental is smaller, which translates into a decreased clearance of the drug. This is thought to be the reason for the delayed awakening after a prolonged infusion of thiopental.

Barbiturates enhance the inhibitory effects of the GABA receptor complex and depress the reticular activating system.

Dose-dependent cardiovascular depression is common after barbiturate administration and results in hypotension secondary to vasodilatation. Reflex tachycardia, probably due to a central vagolytic effect, is often encountered after an induction dose of a barbiturate. When the patient has an inadequate heart rate response (beta blockade, inhibited baroreceptor response), a dramatic fall in blood pressure and cardiac output can occur. Depression of the medullary ventilatory center is dose-dependent and apnea usually follows an induction dose of barbiturates. Tidal volume and respiratory rate are generally decreased. Hiccups, coughing, and muscle movement can be observed but are generally mild. Barbiturates appear to have an antianalgesic effect in some patients and can cause a state of excitement, particularly when given in small doses. Sulfur-containing thiopental can cause histamine release, which may exacerbate asthma in susceptible patients. However, the clinical relevance has not been proved. Care must be taken to avoid extravasation of barbiturates. As with any alkaline substance, injection is painful and can lead to skin necrosis. In addition, thiopental can precipitate when acidic drugs are given simultaneously.

Propofol

Propofol is a rapid and short-acting intravenous anesthetic, which has been evaluated extensively and used for sedation. Due to its favorable pharmacokinetics, propofol can be given as a continuous infusion and one can rapidly achieve different levels of sedation by changing the dose. It is the best hypnotic drug available for administration by continuous infusion. Rapid recovery occurs even after prolonged infusions and recovery is essentially independent of infusion duration. Its high lipid solubility results in a very fast onset (30–60 sec), similar to thiopental, and the drug effect is terminated, after a single bolus, by redistribution. Biotransformation of propofol is exeptionally high (significantly higher than of thiopental). Although conjugated in the liver to inactive metabolites, cirrhosis does not seem to alter the pharmacokinetic properties of propofol. In part, this might be secondary to extrahepatic clearance of propofol, which must exist because propofol's clearance exceeds hepatic blood flow.

Similar to the benzodiazepines, propofol's mechanism of action appears to involve the GABA receptor complex and its hypnotic effect is dose-dependent. The effects on different organ systems are dose-dependent and fairly predictable. Propofol decreases blood pressure because it decreases systemic vascular resistance and decreases myocardial contractility. Heart rate is not significantly altered with the administration of propofol, which suggests that the baroreceptor reflex is inhibited, preventing an increased heart rate response to the lowered blood pressure. Like all hypnotics, propofol can cause significant respiratory depression and apnea after a standard induction dose for anesthesia. Of note is that even at levels used for conscious sedation, the respiratory drive is depressed despite the elevation in carbon dioxide and the decrease in oxygen levels. Upper airway reflexes can be profoundly inhibited with airway obstruction occurring frequently. A beneficial effect of propofol is that it has antiemetic properties at low doses. Currently two formulations of propofol are available in the U.S.; the generic form of propofol contains sulfites, which can cause bronchospasm in susceptible individuals. Furthermore, the emulsion in propofol contains egg phosphatide, which also can cause allergic reactions in susceptible patients. Furthermore, the intravenous injection of propofol often causes pain and irritation of the injected vein. Administering a small dose of local anesthetic (e.g., lidocaine) prior to propofol administration can attenuate this effect.

Ketamine

Ketamine is a structural analogue of phencyclidine (PCP); this is the reason ketamine may cause dysphoria. Ketamine is different from other hypnotic drugs because it has significant analgesic properities. It can be given intravenously or intramuscularly. Even after intramuscular injection, peak plasma levels are achieved after 10–15 minutes. Termination of its effect after a single dose is due to redistribution away from the site of action. Ketamine is metabolized in the liver to several metabolites. Norketamine, one of the metabolites, has been shown to have anesthetic activity, although substantially less than the parent compound. Ketamine has a high hepatic extraction ratio, indicating that metabolism of ketamine is hepatic blood flow-dependent. The mechanism of action is complex and probably involves the thalamus, cortex, and limbic system. Depression of certain parts of the brain and simultaneous stimulation of others create a state that is named dissociative anesthesia. Patients who receive ketamine appear to be awake, their eyes are open and gazing. In fact, it resembles a cataleptic state in that patients have no recollection and are unable to respond to external stimuli. As mentioned, ketamine also provides profound analgesia. Unlike other hypnotic agents, ketamine does not compromise the cardiovascular system. Indeed, it produces an increase in heart rate and blood pressure in a dose-dependent manner. While this might be desirable in a certain patient population (e.g., trauma), health care providers need to understand that these effects can be detrimental in patients with coronary artery disease or hypertension. In clinically relevant doses respiratory depression is minimal to modest and upper airway skeletal muscle tone is well maintained. In fact, ketamine is advocated by some clinicians for patients with asthma or obstructive airway disease, since it supposedly relaxes bronchial smooth muscle. Increased salivation after ketamine administration can be offset by premedication with an anticholinergic agent.

Ketamine should not be administered to patients with increased intracranial pressure as it has negative effects on cerebral oxygen consumption and on cerebral blood flow; however, patients with clinically increased intracranial pressure should not undergo conscious sedation in the first place. One of the most undesirable side effects of ketamine is its psychomimetic profile (e.g., unpleasant dreams, dysphoria). These side effects occur mainly during emergence and during recovery, and can last as long as 24 hours; these problems are more prominent in adults compared to children. Premedication with benzodiazepines has been shown to favorably influence these unwanted side effects. One of the indications for ketamine is an uncooperative patient without intravenous access who has to be sedated. In most cases, intramuscular injections result in adequate conditions for intravenous line placements and for beginning a procedure. However, it needs to be kept in mind that a state of dissociative anesthesia has been induced and aspiration and loss of the airway still can occur.

References

1. Collins VJ (ed): Physiologic and Pharmacologic Bases of Anesthesia. Baltimore, Williams & Wilkins, 1996.
2. Epstein BS: Role of the Anesthesiologist in Analgesia-Sedation; How, When, and Where? Refresher Courses in Anesthesiology, Vol. 25, Chapter 4, 1997.
3. Fragen RJ (ed): Drug Infusion in Anesthesiology, 2nd ed. Philadelphia, Lippincott-Raven, 1996.
4. Goodman LS, Limbird LE, Molinoff PB, Gilman AG (eds): Goodman & Gilman's The Pharmacological Basis of Therapeutics, 9th ed. New York, McGraw-Hill, 1996.
5. Longnecker DE, Murphy FL (eds): Introduction to Anesthesia, 8th ed. Philadelphia, W.B. Saunders, 1992.
6. Miller RD (editor): Anesthesia, 4th ed. New York, Churchill Livingstone, 1994.
7. Sa Rego MM, Watcha MF, White PF: The changing role of monitored anesthesia care in the ambulatory setting. Anesth Analg 85:1020–1036, 1997.

2

Reversal of Conscious Sedation

C. Spencer Yost, M.D.

An important class of drugs that complement those used for conscious sedation are agents that reverse or antagonize the actions of sedative drugs. These compounds allow a patient's sensorium and protective reflexes to be restored quickly to their pre-sedation state. In an era of cost-conscious medicine, a rapid return to normalcy can be cost-effective, saving time spent in a recovery unit or in the emergency department. More importantly, reversal agents may be life-saving if a patient is unexpectedly sensitive to a given sedative/hypnotic drug.

Fortunately, reliable agents are available that can rapidly and safely overcome the depressive effects of most commonly used sedative drugs. This chapter reviews the physiology and pharmacology of agents that can reverse the action of drugs used for sedation. However, not every drug, including some of the most popular currently used drugs, has a specific antagonist. There is also nonspecific reversal that may have occasional use and this also is reviewed here. Nonetheless, having the ability to block the action of an administered sedative drug does not relieve the clinician from the responsibility of abiding by the principles for the safe administration of sedative agents outlined in other chapters of this book.

Pharmacologic Concepts

Almost all drugs produce their desired clinical effect at low concentration in a tissue. They do so by binding to a specific molecular site in a protein, thereby causing a desired change in cellular function and in the tissue that the cells comprise. The binding site is said to have a high affinity for the drug, i.e., the drug is embraced strongly by molecular forces within the protein structure. Binding then leads to a conformational change in the binding protein that alters its activity.

The idea that discrete cellular proteins can "receive" inputs from a source external to the cell to produce a physiologic effect is over a hundred years old. Specific integral membrane proteins that mediate the receptor function have

TABLE 1. Receptor Systems

Receptor	Physiologic Type	Drugs	Reversal Drugs
Opioid	G protein–coupled	Morphine Opioids	Naloxone Nalmefene
GABA$_A$/BZR	Ligand-gated	Benzodiazepines	Flumazenil
GABA$_A$	Ligand-gated	Barbiturates Etomidate Propofol Volatile anesthetics	Physostigmine (?)
NMDA receptor	Ligand-gated	Ketamine	Physostigmine (?)
Nicotinic AChR (neuronal)	Ligand-gated	–	Physostigmine (?)
Muscarinic AChR	G protein–coupled	Atropine	Physostigmine (?)

GABA, gamma-aminobutyric acid; BZR, benzodiazepine receptor; AChR, acetylcholine receptor; NMDA, N-methyl-D-aspartate.

now been isolated and the DNA sequences coding for them have been cloned. These cloned receptors provide tangible, molecular proof for the concept of cellular proteins that act as binding sites for drugs.

Binding of a drug to a receptor is the first step in a pharmacologic response. An agonist drug binds to the receptor, producing a cellular response characteristic for its effect. An antagonist blocks or inhibits the cellular pharmacologic effect. Antagonists can be of two types: (1) competitive antagonists, whose molecular structure is similar to the agonist, allowing them to compete for binding at the high-affinity site; (2) noncompetitive antagonists, which cause inhibition by binding at a site distant from the agonist binding site. Oftentimes, for ion channels, noncompetitive antagonists block the conducting pathway for ion permeation, preventing open channels from conducting current; therefore, increasing concentrations of agonist can overcome competitive inhibition by "out-competing" the inhibiting drug, but they cannot overcome noncompetitive inhibition because functional inhibition occurs at a place on the receptor not involved in agonist binding.

Table 1 lists the receptors that are the primary targets of drugs used in anesthesia and that may be manipulated for conscious sedation. Opioids are a group of drugs that are opium- or morphine-like in the effect they produce. Opioid receptors are members of a structural class with a conserved seven transmembrane structure. These receptors interact with (are coupled to) a family of cellular mediators known as G proteins, which produce a change in cellular function by activating intracellular effector systems such as protein kinases, ion channels, or Ca^{++} storage compartments. The ultimate effector after stimulation of the transmembrane receptor is cell-specific. Therefore, opioids have pleuripotent cellular effects, depending on the type of linkage made by the transducer elements (G proteins) to cellular pathways in a particular tissue. Opioids produce potent relief of pain that also may be accompanied by a central sedative quality and depression of respiratory drive. Several antagonist drugs are available that specifically reverse the action of opioids.

The $GABA_A$ receptor belongs to another large class of receptors known as ligand-gated ion channels (see Tanelian et al.[25] for a review). The $GABA_A$ family is activated by the neurotransmitter gamma-aminobutyric acid (GABA) and selectively passes chloride ions (Cl^-) from the extracellular space to the intracellular side of the membrane, thereby hyperpolarizing the neuronal membrane. This hyperpolarization makes the neuronal cell more resistant to depolarizing influences, preventing action potential propagation. Several different sedative drugs, including benzodiazepines, barbiturates, steroid anesthetics, propofol, ethanol, and volatile anesthetics have enhancing effects on $GABA_A$ receptors and probably mediate their clinical effects through enhanced $GABA_A$ activity. As discussed below, only the action of benzodiazepines on this class of receptor can be specifically antagonized.

Other receptor systems listed in Table 1 may have roles in producing the deepest state of sedation, i.e., general anesthesia. In the case of volatile general anesthetics, a specific receptor system that exclusively mediates the hypnotic action of these drugs has not been identified.

The primary agents discussed in this review are those that reverse the effects of opioids and benzodiazepines. An important feature of the pharmacology of these two classes of agents is their tendency to produce tolerance and dependence. Tolerance can be defined as the need, during chronic drug exposure, for increasing amounts of drug to produce the same therapeutic effect. Dependence is defined as the tendency for a drug to produce a physical and/or psychological withdrawal syndrome upon discontinuation of the drug. Opioids show a much greater potential for tolerance than do the benzodiazepines; during a course of chronic opioid use, the effective dose can increase 100- to 1000-fold.[8] Opioid withdrawal is also generally more severe, manifesting with vomiting, diarrhea, dizziness, tremulousness, and in its severest form with seizures and pulmonary edema. Withdrawal from benzodiazepines generally produces symptoms of anxiety, tremulousness, headache, tinnitus, and insomnia.

The phenomena of tolerance and withdrawal are important aspects of pharmacology to consider when contemplating the use of reversal drugs. Far greater amount of reversal drugs may be needed in drug-tolerant patients.

Furthermore, rapid antagonism of a chronically used agent may precipitate a severe withdrawal crisis.

Reversal of Opioids

Opioid receptors have been the target of natural painkiller substances for thousands of years. The existence of analgesic pathways that can be exogenously stimulated suggested that there may be endogenous substances that stimulate the same pathways. The discovery of enkephalins, endorphins, and dynorphins in the 1970s confirmed this hypothesis. And just as there are varieties of endogenous agonists, there are also varieties of receptors that bind opioids. Opioid receptor subtypes (μ, δ, and κ) represent transmembrane receptors with different amino acid sequences, which translate into small but significant differences in agonist binding site. Consequently, receptor subtypes differ with respect to the drugs to which they respond and to the cellular effect that they produce in the tissues that express them. Opioids are used as adjuvants to local anesthetics and to hypnotic drugs during conscious sedation. However, they do not provide reliable sedation without ventilatory depression when used alone for conscious sedation. Respiratory depression is also much more likely when opioids are combined with other sedative drugs.

Naloxone is a competitive narcotic antagonist used in the management and reversal of overdoses caused by opioids. Unlike some mixed antagonists, which do not completely inhibit the analgesic properties of opiates, naloxone antagonizes all actions of morphine. It also effectively competes with high affinity for binding at all three subtypes of opioid receptor (μ, δ, and κ).[28]

The onset of action of naloxone occurs within 2 minutes; the duration of action is 30-60 minutes. Administration of naloxone is indicated for the complete or partial reversal of CNS and respiratory depression induced by opioids. The following narcotic agonists can be antagonized by naloxone: morphine sulfate, heroin, dilaudid, methadone, meperidine, paregoric, fentanyl citrate, oxycodone (Percodan), codeine, propoxyphene (Darvon). The depressive effects of mixed agonist/antagonist such as butorphanol tartrate (Stadol), pentazocine (Talwin), nalbuphine (Nubain) and buprenorphine (Buprenex) can also be reversed by naloxone.

The primary indication for the administration of naloxone is decreased level of consciousness especially accompanied by respiratory depression. As opioid compounds have potent inhibitory effects on respiratory centers, hypoventilation and desaturation are known side effects of these agents. Naloxone rapidly reverses this depression.

Less clear is the role of naloxone for treatment of coma of unknown origin in patients presenting to an emergency room (ER). Hoffman and Goldfrank

TABLE 2. Half-Lives of Opioids and Antagonists

Generic Name	Brand Name	Half-Life
Opioid		
Morphine		2–3 hrs
Meperidine	Demerol	2–4 hrs
Fentanyl	Sublimaze	α = 15 min, β = 3 hrs
Sufentanil	Sufenta	α = 15 min, β = 2 hrs
Alfentanil	Alfenta	α = 10 min, β = 90 min
Remifentanil	Ultiva	3–6 min
Butorphanol	Stadol	2.5–3.5 hrs
Nalbuphine	Nubain	5 hrs
Antagonist		
Naloxone	Narcan	30–60 min
Naltrexone	Trexan	4–10 hrs
Nalmefene	Revex	11 hrs

reviewed the use of emergency room treatment of patients with altered consciousness and formulated a consensus treatment regimen based on large published trials.[11] Naloxone is widely used as part of the "coma cocktail," along with oxygen, hypertonic dextrose, and thiamine for the empiric treatment of patients with altered consciousness. Ideally, however, administration of naloxone should only occur when signs of opioids are present.

The need to reverse conscious sedation with naloxone in pediatric populations appears to be low. Graff et al. studied 339 children aged 1–18 years of age in the ER requiring sedation for reduction of fractures and dislocations.[5] Sedation was accomplished with fentanyl/midazolam with an average dose of 1.5 µg/kg for fentanyl and 0.17 mg/kg for midazolam. The primary complication was respiratory depression in 5–10% and most were managed with simple reminders to breathe, airway positioning and/or supplemental oxygen. Only two out of 339 patients had respiratory depression serious enough to require administration of naloxone.

The adverse reactions associated with the administration of naloxone include tachycardia, hypertension, dysrhythmias, nausea, vomiting and diaphoresis. A rare but serious side effect that has been reported is seizure but no causal relationship has been established. Naloxone should not be given to patients with known allergic hypersensitivity to the drug unless life-threatening respiratory depression is present. It should also be used with caution in narcotic-dependent patients who may experience a withdrawal syndrome, including neonates of narcotic-dependent mothers. Caution also should be be exercised when administering naloxone to chronic opioid users or abusers as it may precipitate withdrawal with hypertension, tachycardia, pulmonary edema and violent behavior. Naloxone is not recommended for use in pregnant women because of the lack of information about the effects of the drug on the unborn fetus. Also, naloxone should not be used in nursing mothers because it is not known if the drug is excreted in the mother's milk.

Naloxone is supplied in three different strengths: 0.02 mg/ml (20 µg/ml) (neonate), 0.4 mg/ml (400 µg/ml), and 1 mg/ml. The published guidelines for adult dosing generally fall into two categories: low-dose and high-dose. High dosing is usually used in the ER setting to reverse patients with severe respiratory depression or apnea with or without known opioid use: 0.4–2 mg intravenously, intramuscularly, or subcutaneously. The most rapid effect is seen with intravenous dosing. These doses may be repeated at 5-minute intervals to a maximum of 10 mg. Low-end dosing calls for titration of small doses, usually 40-µg boluses, that are repeated frequently (every minute) until an increased respiratory rate is observed or the patient wakes up. Patients who are hypoventilating and with low oxygen saturations should have assisted ventilation by bag-mask system or endotracheal intubation with supplemental oxygen during the administration of naloxone. For pediatric patients naloxone should be given at a dose of 0.1 mg/kg/dose intravenously, intramuscularly, or subcutaneously; if no response is observed in 10 minutes, administer an additional 0.1 mg/kg/dose. The recommended intravenous dose of nalmefene is 0.25 µg/kg repeated every 2–3 minutes up to a total dose of 1 µg/kg.[21]

A significant drawback to the use of naloxone in patient who have received opioids is its short half-life. Table 2 lists commonly used opioids and their half-lives along with the useful antagonists and their half-lives. Naltrexone and nalmefene are long-acting opioid antagonists. These long-lasting antagonists may have a role in managing side effects of opioid treatment. For example, Yuan et al. administered methylnaltrexone to patients on methadone treatment and were able to reverse constipation in the study group, reducing oral-cecal transit time by 77 minutes, a statistically significant difference.[31] Naloxone also may aid colonoscopic examinations by enhancing the appearance of the colon vasculature and of colonic vascular ectasias.[3]

Occasionally, reversal of respiratory depression is required in hospitalized patients who have been given opioids for postoperative pain control, but the incidence appears low. Scott et al. studied the incidence of respiratory depression in patients on an acute pain service who had received bupivacaine/fentanyl epidurally. Only four of these 1,014 patients had respiratory depression necessitating naloxone treatment.[23] Tsui et al. examined the need for reversal in patients on an acute pain service. Two patients out of over 2500 required the administration of naloxone for bradyapnea and/or desaturation.[26]

Naloxone and its longer-lasting relative nalmefene represent important intravenous agents that must be readily available any time opioids are administered during conscious sedation. These drugs also have life-saving potential in ER and hospital ward settings

Reversal of Benzodiazepines

The target of benzodiazepines is a transmembrane protein complex that functions as a ligand-gated ion channel activated by the neurotransmitter GABA. $GABA_A$ receptor family members are comprised of multiple subunits; the inclusion of one specific subunit, the $\gamma2$ subunit, in the multimeric complex is a requisite for benzodiazepine binding and enhancement of its Cl^- current. $GABA_A$ receptors containing the $\gamma2$ subunit are termed benzodiazepine receptors and probably represent the most widely expressed form of GABA receptor in the central nervous system.

Flumazenil, an imidazobenzodiazepine, is a benzodiazepine antagonist that blocks, by competitive inhibition, the central effects of agents acting via the benzodiazepine receptor. The antagonism is specific, since in animal experiments the effects of compounds that have no affinity for the benzodiazepine receptor (e.g., barbiturates, ethanol, GABA-mimetics) were not affected by flumazenil.[16] Following the intravenous administration of radiolabeled flumazenil to human volunteers, the distribution of radioactivity corresponded closely to the distribution of benzodiazepine receptors as determined by positron emission tomography and could be displaced by administration of midazolam.[17]

The hypnotic-sedative effects of benzodiazepines are rapidly reversed by flumazenil. The trade name of flumazenil is Romazicon; it was formally named Mazicon, but was changed because of confusion with similar-sounding medications. Flumazenil is given intravenously to antagonize sedation, impaired recall, impaired psychomotor function, and respiratory depression in patients who have been given benzodiazepines such as midazolam, valium, flunitrazepam, or lorazepam for sedation or general anesthesia. Quantitative electroencephalographic recordings show that slow wave increases associated with sedation that are induced by benzodiazepines are specifically antagonized by flumazenil.[1,4] The onset of action is rapid with reversal of sedative effects evident within 1–2 minutes. The peak effect occurs within 6–10 minutes. Doses of 0.1–0.2 mg produce peak plasma levels of 3–6 ng/ml that are associated with partial antagonism of conscious sedation. Doses of 0.4–1.0 mg have peak plasma levels of 12–28 ng/ml, which usually produces complete competitive antagonism of sedation. For reversal of general anesthesia state produced by benzodiazepines the recommended initial dose is 0.2 mg administered intravenously over 15 seconds. If the desired level of consciousness is not obtained within 60 seconds, a further dose of 0.1 mg can be injected and repeated at 60-second intervals, up to a maximum total dose of 1 mg. The usual dose is between 0.3 and 0.6 mg.

The ability of flumazenil to reverse benzodiazepine-induced respiratory depression is equivocal; in some studies residual effects of benzodiazepines on respiration were still present despite reversal of sedation.[19] The ability of flumazenil to reverse respiratory depression caused by a combination of benzodiazepine and opioids—a commonly used combination of agents used for conscious sedation—has also been called into question by a number of studies. To study this issue, Gross et al. used normal volunteers to induce respiratory depression and assessed the ability of flumazenil to reverse ventilatory depression produced by the combination of an opioid (alfentanil) and midazolam.[6] Respiratory depression was produced incrementally first by the opioid, then by the benzodiazepine, as measured by slope of the CO_2 response curve and by the minute ventilation at pCO_2 = 50 mmHg. In this study flumazenil (1 mg load, 20 µg/min infusion) effectively reversed the respiratory depression component due to midazolam. Therefore, when used at the end of anesthesia, flumazenil should not be given until the effects of neuromuscular blockade have been completely antagonized and careful monitoring of the respiratory depressant effect of opiate analgesics has been assured. After the benzodiazepine has been antagonized with flumazenil, any residual respiratory depressant effect of other agents, such as opiates, should be appropriately treated.[13] In addition, postoperative pain must be taken into account. Following a major surgery, it may be preferable to maintain a moderate degree of sedation.

The half-life of flumazenil is 7–15 minutes and it is removed from the circulation by a combination of redistribution and metabolism. Flumazenil is metabolized in the liver to a water-soluble inactive form and excreted by the kidneys. In patients with cirrhosis, the pharmacokinetics of flumazenil is altered, particularly in patients with severely impaired liver function. Flumazenil undergoes rapid and extensive hepatic metabolism; less than 0.2% of the administered dose is eliminated unchanged in the urine. The major metabolites of flumazenil identified in the urine are the free acid and its glucuronide conjugate. In healthy volunteers, approximately 70% of an intravenous dose of flumazenil is excreted within the first 2 hours after dosing and another 16% during the next 2 hours. Elimination was essentially complete within 72 hours, with 90–95% of the total radioactivity appearing in the urine and 5–10% in the feces. Therefore, elimination half-life is prolonged and plasma clearance markedly decreased in cirrhotic patients with limited drug-metabolizing hepatic reserve.

Plasma protein binding is rather low. Over a concentration range of 24–570 ng/ml, flumazenil was found to be 50% bound to human plasma proteins. Albumin accounts for approximately two-thirds of the plasma protein binding. The binding of flumazenil was not affected by a high concentration of diazepam

(10 µg/ml), and flumazenil did not interfere with the binding of diazepam. When administered together with the benzodiazepine midazolam, the pharmacokinetic parameters of flumazenil were not affected. Similarly, the pharmacokinetics of benzodiazepines remained unaltered in the presence of the antagonist flumazenil. Since plasma protein binding is lower in cirrhotic patients than in healthy subjects, the levels of free drug are also substantially increased, namely from 55% in controls to 64% and 79% in patients with moderate and severe liver dysfunction, respectively.

In patients with chronic stabilized renal failure (creatinine clearance < 10 ml/min) in the absence and presence of dialysis, the pharmacokinetics of flumazenil remained essentially unaltered. Thus, no dosage adjustments are necessary in patients with renal impairment.

Flumazenil is generally well tolerated. In postoperative use, nausea and/or vomiting may be observed, particularly if opiates have also been used. Flushing has also been noted. If patients are awakened too rapidly, CNS symptoms such as startle reaction, nervousness, restlessness, excitation, aggressiveness, anger, euphoria, hallucinations, vertigo, confusion, drowsiness, depression, tremor, or tetany may occur and they may become agitated, anxious, or fearful. Transient increases in blood pressure and heart rate also may occur. Excessive or too rapidly injected doses of flumazenil may induce benzodiazepine withdrawal symptoms such as anxiety attacks, tachycardia, dizziness, and sweating in patients on long-term benzodiazepine treatment. Cardiovascular side effects in these circumstances include ventricular premature beats, arrhythmia, palpitations, bradycardia, flush, and hypotension. Seizures and/or severe cardiac arrhythmias have been observed in patients who are physically dependent on benzodiazepines. Administration of flumazenil is contraindicated in persons with a known hypersensitivity to flumazenil or to benzodiazepines.

However, the residual effects of sedation may reappear gradually within a few hours after conscious sedation, depending on the dose of flumazenil, the time elapsed since the benzodiazepine agonist was given, and the dose and elimination half-life of the previously administered benzodiazepine. The mean elimination half-life of flumazenil following the administration of single intravenous dose to healthy subjects was approximately 1 hour. Therefore, as with naloxone, there is a possibility that benzodiazepine reversal may decrease within an hour and resedation could occur. Even though psychomotor function can be fully restored with flumazenil (tested in one study by P-deletion, choice reaction time, and Maddox wing tests), conservative guidelines for return to normal activities should probably be followed.[14] In a U.S. clinical study in patients with benzodiazepine intoxication, 90/133 patients (67.7%) became resedated. In view of the short duration of action of flumazenil and the possible need for repeat doses, the patient should remain closely monitored until all possible central benzodiazepine effects have subsided. Therefore, flumazenil should be administered only when the continued observation of patients for recurrence of sedation can be assured. Upon discharge from a conscious sedation setting, patients who have received flumazenil to reverse the effects of benzodiazepine sedation should be instructed, if possible in writing, not to drive, to operate machinery, or to engage in any other physically or mentally demanding activity for 24 hours or until the effects of the benzodiazepine have subsided, since the effects may return. Patients should also be warned not to take alcohol or drugs not prescribed by their physician until the effects of the benzodiazepines have subsided.

Flumazenil may also have application as part of the "coma cocktail" but it is probably best reserved for the reversal of therapeutic sedation and for the occasional known benzodiazepine overdose.[29] Incremental intravenous doses of 0.1–0.3 mg can be effective in diagnosis and treating pure benzodiazepine overdose in adults. The intravenous dose in children is 5–10 µg/kg. In cases of known or suspected benzodiazepine overdose, titrate flumazenil until the patient clearly responds or until the maximum recommended dose has been reached. The recommended initial dose is 0.3 mg administered intravenously over 30 seconds, followed by a series of 0.3 mg injections, each administered over a 30-second period at 60-second intervals. The maximum recommended dose is 2.0 mg. If a significant improvement in the level of consciousness and respiratory function is not achieved after repeated injections of flumazenil, a non-benzodiazepine etiology must be assumed. If drowsiness recurs, an intravenous infusion of 0.1–0.4 mg/hr may be useful. The rate of the infusion should be individually adjusted to the desired level of arousal.

However, flumazenil must be used with caution in multiple drug overdoses, in patients with alcoholism, and patients with other drug dependencies. Since flumazenil abruptly terminates the effects of benzodiazepines, sympathetic tone may be suddenly increased and, thus, cardiac electrical instability enhanced. Consequently, caution is advised when administering flumazenil to patients with myocardial infarction or cardiac arrhythmias. Particular caution is necessary when using flumazenil in cases of multiple drug overdose, since the toxic effects (cardiac arrhythmias and/or convulsions) of other psychotropic drugs, especially tricyclic antidepressants, may increase as the effects of benzodiazepines subside. Patients should be specifically evaluated for the signs and symptoms of a tricyclic antidepressant overdose. A diagnostic ECG can be used to confirm the presence of these agents; a QRS duration of 0.1 seconds or greater indicates a serious overdosage with tricyclic antidepressants, which should be treated with appropriate measures. Depending on the extent of involvement of benzodiazepines in the multiple drug overdose, this may or may not include flumazenil.

Special consideration should be used when administering flumazenil in certain specific clinical situations. The dosage of flumazenil should be adjusted carefully in patients suffering from preoperative anxiety or having a history of chronic or episodic anxiety. In anxious patients, particularly those with coronary artery disease, it may be preferable to maintain a degree of sedation throughout the early post-sedation period rather than bring about complete arousal. Flumazenil is contraindicated in epileptic patients who have been receiving benzodiazepine treatment for a prolonged period. The abrupt suppression of the protective effect of benzodiazepines may induce convulsions in epileptic patients. Finally, there are no adequate and well-controlled studies of the use of flumazenil in pregnant women, therefore flumazenil should be used during pregnancy only if the potential benefit justifies the potential risk to the fetus.

The safety and effectiveness of flumazenil in children below the age of 18 has not been fully established. Two studies have indicated that flumazenil is well tolerated by children for reversal of conscious sedation with either midazolam or diazepam.[20,24] However, a shortening of the recovery period could not be demonstrated with the routine use of flumazenil and resedation occurred in 8%, primarily in the youngest age group (1–5 years).

In the absence of data on the use of flumazenil in elderly patients, it should be borne in mind that this population is generally more sensitive to the effects of sedative drugs; flumazenil has been used after bronchoscopy with good effect to improve breathing and oxygen saturation.[30] It is not known whether flumazenil is excreted in human milk. For this reason, breastfeeding should be interrupted for 24 hours when flumazenil is used during lactation.

Flumazenil has shown some weak intrinsic agonistic (e.g., anticonvulsant) activity without therapeutic relevance. However, this minor agonist potential may have a role in ameliorating benzodiazepine withdrawal symptoms. Saxon et al. used a double-blind, placebo-controlled cross-over study design to determine if flumazenil could reduce symptoms of withdrawal in benzodiazepine-dependent patients.[22] They found a small reduction in the negative feelings that were attributable to benzodiazepine withdrawal.

Flumazenil is to be used by intravenous administration only. It is available in multidose vials of 5 ml/0.1 mg/ml or 10 ml/0.1 mg/ml. This drug should have no ceiling, but total dose given should not exceed 1–2 mg. Flumazenil may be diluted with sodium chloride 0.9%, sodium chloride 0.45% + dextrose 2.5%, or dextrose 5% for infusion. Infusion solutions are stable for up to 24 hours when stored at room temperature.

In summary, the dose of flumazenil should always be individually titrated to the desired response to avoid abrupt awakening. Particular care is needed with patients who are physically dependent on benzodiazepines, patients who have ingested multiple drugs, and patients who are prone to anxiety.

Nonspecific Reversal

Opioid and benzodiazepine reversal agents discussed above produce rapid, specific antagonism of drugs used in conscious sedation by acting directly on known receptor systems. Another agent, physostigmine, has also shown the ability to "reverse" sedation, i.e., cause an unconscious, unresponsive patient to wake up, follow commands, and have intact airway reflexes. Physostigmine has been reported to reverse sedation produced by a large number of different agents, suggesting a nonspecific, probably noncompetitive type of antagonism through other pathways. The fact that physostigmine can cross the blood–brain barrier and inhibit acetylcholinesterase in the central nervous system indicates that enhancement of central cholinergic pathways is the likely mechanism by which physostimine causes reversal of sedation.

Holzgrafe et al. first reported the use of physostimine for reversal of the sedative effects of scopolamine in 1973.[10] They reported that sedation produced by the anti-muscarinic agent scopolomine could be antagonized by physostigmine. Later investigators expanded the list of sedative drugs that physostigmine can reverse. The sedative effects of drugs as diverse as barbiturates, benzodiazepines, nitrous oxide, cimetidine, enflurane, isoflurane, halothane, and ketamine have been reversed by physostigmine.[2,7,9,10,15,18] Animal studies in dogs and rodents have confirmed that physostimine has centrally activating ability.[12]

The mechanism by which physostimine nonspecifically reverses sedation is not established but it presumably involves stimulation of cholinergic neurons critically for attention and cortical activation.[18,27] These neuronal networks are located in the septal region and are also the target of drugs, such as tacrine, used to improve mental functioning in Alzheimer's patients. The effective dose of physostigmine is 25 µg/kg (about 2 mg in a 70-kg adult). Signs of peripheral hyperactivity, such as salivation, defecation, miosis, and muscle twitching have been observed in animal studies at high dosages (> 200 µg/kg).[27]

Conclusions

The existence of rapid, specific antagonists of opioids and benzodiazepines provides an important degree of safety during conscious sedation. However, administration of these agents should be undertaken with care as the underlying medical condition of a given patient may greatly influence the incidence of side effects. Nonspecific reversal with physostigmine also appears to be capable of facilitating emergence from variety of different sedating drugs.

References

1. Bonfiglio MF, Fisher-Katz LE, Saltis LM, et al: A pilot pharmacokinetic-pharmacodynamic study of benzodiazepine antagonism by flumazenil and aminophylline. Pharmacotherapy 16:1166–1172, 1996.

2. Bourke DL, Rosenberg M, Allen PD: Physostigmine: Effectiveness as an antagonist of respiratory depression and psychomotor effects caused by morphine or diazepam. Anesthesiology 61:523–528, 1984

3. Brandt LJ, Spinnell MK: Ability of naloxone to enhance the colonoscopic appearance of normal colon vasculature and colon vascular ectasias. Gastrointest Endosc 49:79–83, 1999.

4. Fiset P, Lemmens HL, Egan TE, et al: Pharmacodynamic modeling of the electroencephalographic effects of flumazenil in healthy volunteers sedated with midazolam. Clin Pharmacol Ther 58:567–582, 1995.

5. Graff KJ, Kennedy RM, Jaffe DM: Conscious sedation for pediatric orthopaedic emergencies. Pediatr Emerg Care 12:31–35, 1996.

6. Gross JB, Blouin RT, Zandsberg S, et al: Effect of flumazenil on ventilatory drive during sedation with midazolam and alfentanil. Anesthesiology 85:713–720, 1996.

7. Hamilton-Davies C, Bailie R, Restall J: Physostigmine in recovery from anaesthesia. Anaesthesia 50:456–458, 1995.

8. Harrison LM, Kastin AJ, Zadina JE: Opiate tolerance and dependence: Receptors, G-proteins, and antiopiates. Peptides 19:1603–1630, 1998.

9. Hill GE, Stanley TH, Sentker CR: Physostigmine reversal of postoperative somnolence. Can Anaesth Soc J 24:707–711, 1977.

10. Holzgrafe RE, Vondrell JJ, Mintz SM: Reversal of postoperative reactions to scopolamine with physostigmine. Anesth Analg 52:921–925, 1973.

11. Hoffman RS, Goldfrank LR: The poisoned patient with altered consciousness. Controversies in the use of a "coma cocktail". JAMA 274:562–529, 1995.

12. Horrigan RW: Physostigmine and anesthetic requirement for halothane in dogs. Anesth Analg 57:180–185, 1978.

13. Jensen AG, Moller JT, Lybecker H, Hansen PA: A random trial comparing recovery after midazolam-alfentanil anesthesia with and without reversal with flumazenil, and standardized neuroleptic anesthesia for major gynecologic surgery. J Clin Anesth 7:63–70, 1995.

14. Kankaria A, Lewis JH, Ginsberg G, et al: Flumazenil reversal of psychomotor impairment due to midazolam or diazepam for conscious sedation for upper endoscopy. Gastrointest Endosc 44:416–421, 1996.

15. Kesecioglu J, Rupreht J, Telci L, et al: Effect of aminophylline or physostigmine on recovery from nitrous oxide-enflurane anaesthesia. Acta Anaesthesiol Scand 35:616–620, 1991.

16. Lipartiti M, Arban R, Fadda E, et al: Characterization of [^{3}H]-imidazenil binding to rat brain membranes. Br J Pharmacol 114:1159–1164, 1995.

17. Malizia AL, Gunn RN, Wilson SJ, et al: Benzodiazepine site pharmacokinetic/pharmaco-dynamic quantification in man: Direct measurement of drug occupancy and effects on the human brain in vivo. Neuropharmacology 35:1483–1491, 1996.

18. Martin B, Howell PR: Physostigmine: Going ... going ... gone? Two cases of central anticholinergic syndrome following anaesthesia and its treatment with physostigmine. Eur J Anaesthesiol 14:467–470, 1997.

19. Mora CT, Torjman M, White PF: Sedative and ventilatory effects of midazolam infusion: Effect of flumazenil reversal. Can J Anaesth 42:677–684, 1995.

20. Peters JM, Tolia V, Simpson P, et al: Flumazenil in children after esophagogastroduodenoscopy. Am J Gastroenterol 94:1857–1861, 1999.

21. Sa Rego MM, Watcha MF, White PF: The changing role of monitored anesthesia care in the ambulatory setting. Anesthesiology 85:1020–1036, 1997.

22. Saxon L, Hjemdahl P, Hiltunen AJ, Borg S: Effects of flumazenil in the treatment of benzodiazepine withdrawal: A double-blind pilot study. Psychopharmacology 131: 153–160, 1997.

23. Scott DA, Beilby DS, McClymont C: Postoperative analgesia using epidural infusions of fentanyl with bupivacaine: A prospective analysis of 1,014 patients. Anesthesiology 83:727–737, 1995.

24. Shannon M, Albers G, Burkhart K, et al: Safety and efficacy of flumazenil in the reversal of benzodiazepine-induced conscious sedation: The Flumazenil Pediatric Study Group. J Pediatr 131:582–586, 1997.

25. Tanelian DL, Kosek P, Mody I, MacIver MB: The role of the $GABA_A$ receptor/chloride channel complex in anesthesia. Anesthesiology 78:757–776, 1993.

26. Tsui SL, Irwin MG, Wong CM, et al: An audit of the safety of an acute pain service. Anaesthesia 52:1042–1047, 1997.

27. Vatashsky E, Beilin B, Razin M, Weinstock M: Mechanism of antagonism by physostigmine of acute flunitrazepam intoxication. Anesthesiology 64:248–252, 1986.

28. Wang DS, Sternbach G, Varon J: Nalmefene: A long-acting opioid antagonist. Clinical applications in emergency medicine. J Emerg Med 16:471–475, 1998.

29. Weinbroum AA, Flaishon R, Sorkine P, et al: A risk-benefit assessment of flumazenil in the management of benzodiazepine overdose. Drug Saf 17:181–196, 1997.

30. Williams TJ, Bowie PE: Midazolam sedation to produce complete amnesia for bronchoscopy: 2 years' experience at a district general hospital. Respir Med 93:361–365, 1999.

31. Yuan C-S, Foss JF, O'Connor M, et al: Methylnaltrexone for reversal of constipation due to chronic methadone use. JAMA 283:367–372, 2000.

3

Preprocedure Evaluation for Sedation and Analgesia

Edwin S. Cheng, M.D.
Jeanine P. Wiener-Kronish, M.D.

The preprocedure evaluation is a meeting between the patient and a qualified health practitioner that occurs prior to any procedure requiring sedation and analgesia. This encounter serves several important purposes. The information gathered about the medical status of the patient will guide the practitioner in designing a tailored plan for sedation and analgesia. Preprocedure evaluation allows for the development of a verbal relationship that continues throughout the procedure when verbal communication is critical for assessment of depth of sedation, and concludes at the end of the recovery period. Patients need to have their questions answered regarding the procedure, sedation, and analgesia, thus reducing levels of anxiety and ensuring informed consent.

A thoughtful plan for sedation and analgesia that is the result of an adequate preprocedure evaluation can allow even the patient with marginal reserve to tolerate an unpleasant procedure comfortably and safely. However, the administration of sedative and analgesic drugs without an adequate understanding of the patient's medical problems can lead to catastrophic consequences, including medical-legal problems (see Chapter 12). Therefore, a preprocedural evaluation must always be performed and documentation that it was performed needs to be in the patient's chart.

The Format of the Preprocedure Evaluation

As in a standard preoperative assessment, the preprocedure evaluation consists of the following elements:

1. **A focused medical history:** Information is gathered through a review of the patient's medical chart and the patient interview, usually conducted by a physician or a nurse practitioner.

2. **Physical examination:** A focused examination with particular attention paid to the airway, heart, and lungs not only provides confirmation of an accurate history, but also instills patient confidence in the health care provider and reduces patient anxiety.

3. **Appropriate laboratory tests:** Findings from the history and physical examination may suggest that laboratory or diagnostic testing is prudent. For sedation and analgesia procedures, laboratory testing should only be done if the test results will alter the management of the patient. Routine laboratory screening adds little information already gleaned from an effectively performed history and physical examination. Electrocardiograms should be obtained in patients with any history of cardiac disease or in patients with multiple medical problems (i.e., diabetes, renal failure).

4. **An anesthetic plan:** An assessment of the patient's overall health status then dictates the plan for periprocedural sedation and analgesia, and alternatives for postprocedural analgesia.

5. **Informed consent:** The patient should be informed of the plan, along with the benefits, potential risks and possible side effects of the procedure, and the medications to be used. The patient signs a consent form confirming that the discussion has taken place and that he or she is aware of the risks and agrees to proceed.

The History

The patient's medical history is acquired from two sources—the medical chart and the patient interview. Although the yield of the interview can be maximized if preceded by perusal of the medical chart, the most important information required for a preprocedure evaluation is quickly revealed in the interview. Prior to evaluating the various organ systems, there are general historical items to document, which are essential for the safe administration of sedation and analgesia.

Age

Patients 65 years of age and older often have an increased prevalence of organ dysfunction and medical problems (see Chapter 6). Aging also alters renal and hepatic metabolism so that drug metabolism is changed. Thus, there is an increased chance for prolongation of drug effects. With aging, the central nervous system is more sensitive to the effects of sedatives and analgesics, i.e., anesthesia and sedation are achieved with smaller doses.

Medications

Besides prescription medications, there should be documentation of all ingestions of over-the-counter medications, vitamins, and herbal supplements, as drug interactions can occur. Medications such as the H2-blocker cimetidine inhibit the cytochrome P-450 enzyme system that metabolizes benzodiazepines, leading to prolonged sedation and amnesia in patients receiving both drugs. Similarly, prolonged drug effects are seen in patients taking protease inhibitor drugs routinely given for HIV infection treatment. These drugs include ritonavir, nelfinavir, and saquinavir; they interfere with the metabolism of benzodiazepines and opioids and have been associated with prolonged amnesia.

Allergies

True allergic reactions are immunologically mediated processes that involve antigen–antibody reactions. An example is anaphylaxis, a potentially life-threatening hypersensitivity reaction that results in respiratory obstruction and cardiovascular collapse. A prior history of allergy to a particular drug is an important historical fact that needs to be documented so that the drug can be avoided. Adult patients who report a suspected childhood allergy to penicillin usually may receive cephalosporin antibiotics as a substitute. Patients with allergies to intravenous contrast often receive prophylactic administration of H1- and H2-blocker medications as well as steroids to decrease the allergic reaction. Patients with multiple hospitalizations may develop a dermatologic reaction to adhesive tape. Patients will often confuse a drug reaction (i.e., nausea from codeine ingestion) with a true allergic reaction. Nevertheless, it is prudent practice to avoid administering any medication that is associated with adverse effects and efforts should be made to seek adequate substitutes.

Prior Surgeries, Anesthesia, and Complications from Anesthesia

Anesthetic records from past surgeries or procedures contain valuable information regarding airway management, respiratory and hemodynamic responses to sedation and anesthesia, and postoperative recovery. A documented history of a difficult intubation places the patient at higher risk for complications should airway management become necessary during sedation and analgesia. Prior episodes of hemodynamic instability during sedation or induction may alter pharmacologic management of the patient. Important histories to elicit regarding postoperative complications include the occurrence of nausea and vomiting after sedation or analgesia, and prolonged recovery intervals after sedation.

History of Tobacco Use

A history of tobacco use places the patient in a category of patients at risk for cardiovascular and pulmonary disease. Smoking is an independent risk factor for coronary artery disease. Impaired respiratory function as a result of smoking increases the risk of periprocedural complications, since airway protection and ventilatory responses are depressed by sedation and analgesia. In addition, smoking contributes to increased pulmonary complications in the postoperative period. Although smoking cessation less than 8 weeks prior to the procedure is unlikely to confer any benefit in terms of decreased risk of respiratory complications,[1] the preprocedure evaluation is an important opportunity for the provider to promote smoking cessation as a general means of improving health.

History of Alcohol Use

A history of heavy alcohol intake or alcohol abuse carries several implications for sedative and analgesic management. Long-term alcohol use can be associated with parenchymal liver disease, which will affect the metabolism of drugs. Midazolam, a commonly employed drug for sedation, is metabolized by the liver and its effects will be prolonged in patients with cirrhosis. However, chronic alcohol ingestion in patients who do not yet have cirrhosis is associated with the induction of hepatic enzymes resulting in increased clearance of midazolam. Therefore, it is essential to know whether a patient has liver disease.

Alcohol use also is associated with a number of cardiac and pulmonary conditions, including dilated cardiomyopathy, arrhythmias, coronary artery disease, stroke, hypertension, and respiratory distress syndrome.[4] Also, a high percentage of alcoholics smoke, with as many as 20% of these patients having chronic obstructive pulmonary disease. Patients who ingest alcohol prior to the administration of sedation or analgesia may have a prolonged recovery period due to the ethanol, and also have an increased incidence of delirium when they require hospitalization.

History of Substance Abuse

When encountering the patient with a history of substance abuse or tolerance to opiates, several issues require further questioning and investigation. Accurate determination of the quantity of narcotics used can provide an indication of the amount of analgesics that will be necessary to adequately treat pain and discomfort. In fact, it may be prudent to use drugs other than narcotics for sedation in these patients, as they will be tolerant to all narcotic drugs. Patients on methadone maintenance therapy should be encouraged to continue their regimen prior to the procedure.

The provider must maintain a heightened awareness of the possibility that such a patient may withdraw and become ill, particularly if there is 24–48-hour hiatus before the next ingestion or administration of narcotics. Intravenous drug users present special problems in that intravenous access is often difficult, and they often have other diseases, including hepatitis B and C. Therefore, these patients will be tolerant to narcotics, but if they develop cirrhosis from their hepatitis, their metabolism of these drugs becomes abnormal and they ultimately may only tolerate smaller doses.

Review of Systems

Evaluation of the patient's medical history attempts to ensure that the patient's health is optimized prior to the procedure. Questions should be asked regarding conditions that could compromise patient safety during the administration of sedation and analgesia.

Airways

Although the most valuable information about the airway comes from the physical examination, there are important historical items that, if present, increase the possibility of difficult airway management.

Sleep Apnea. A history of snoring or sleep apnea, defined as cessation of air movement despite ventilatory efforts, can indicate an atypical airway. Sleep apnea is an important condition to inquire about because the anatomy that predisposes to snoring and obstruction of air movement (narrow airways, tonsillar hypertrophy, craniofacial skeletal abnormalities) is also the anatomy that makes the delivery of positive-pressure ventilation using a mask difficult and may also signify that endotracheal intubation will be difficult. Furthermore, sedating patients who have sleep apnea is associated with an increased risk of airway obstruction from the collapse of often ponderous pharyngeal soft tissue. Also, patients who have sleep apnea also have higher rates of cardiovascular disease, including hypertension, pulmonary hypertension, cardiac arrhythmias, myocardial ischemia and infarction, and stroke. Finally, patients with sleep apnea are also more sensitive to sedation, and experience prolonged sedation with the "usual" dosages of sedatives.

Rheumatoid Arthritis or Degenerative Joint Disease. Patients with severe rheumatoid arthritis are at risk for developing airway obstruction as a result of narcotics or sedatives. In addition, they often present with airway anatomy that makes tracheal intubation difficult, and cervical spine instability that may result in spinal cord trauma from manipulation of the neck. Therefore, either an anesthesiologist should be involved with the sedation or drug administration should be closely monitored so that airway obstruction does not occur.

Abnormalities of the Oropharynx. In addition to systemic medical conditions that affect airway management, specific information about the condition of the mouth, jaw, and neck should be reviewed. The presence of removable dental prostheses such as dentures, plates, and bridges or a history of dental cosmetic surgery should be documented, as should any limitations in mouth opening or neck extension. Conditions that preclude endotracheal intubation (inability to open mouth, inability to see pharynx, neck immobility) should alert the practioner that an anesthesiologist should be consulted or be involved in the procedure.

TABLE 1. Possible Preprocedure Cardiac Assessment Tests

Test	Result
Electrocardiogram	Arrhythmias, left ventricular hypertrophy, exercise stress-induced ischemia
Echocardiogram	Ventricular dysfunction, valvular heart disease, prior myocardial infarction
Radionuclide tests	Ejection fraction, reversible perfusion defects
Coronary angiography	Revascularization, valvular disease, wall motion abnormalities

Cardiovascular Abnormalities

With cardiovascular disease being the leading cause of death in the United States as well as a leading contributor to perioperative morbidity and mortality, many of the studies and articles on preoperative evaluation justifiably have focused on assessing and reducing the cardiac-related risk of surgery. Sedation and analgesia usually are given for procedures that are associated with a low risk of cardiac morbidity (myocardial ischemia, infarction, or death). However, patients with a history of unstable angina, new angina, recent myocardial infarctions, or hemodynamic instability are not reasonable candidates for sedation and analgesia for elective procedures. Other cardiac problems that need to be treated maximally prior to elective procedures include congestive heart failure, symptomatic arrhythmias, and major valvular abnormalities. The presence of any of these conditions require further evaluation either for diagnostic purposes or for treatment prior to the procedure.

In the setting of sedation and analgesia, a useful assessment of the cardiovascular condition is based on an estimation of the functional status of the patient. Questions should focus on the presence and duration of any symptoms associated with specific activities, such as:

1. Can you walk one or two city blocks without stopping?
2. Can you climb a flight of stairs or walk up a hill?
3. Can you carry a bag of groceries up the stairs without shortness of breath or chest pain?
4. Can you participate in strenuous sports like swimming, jogging, or skiing?

These questions assess functional capacity, and correlate with the ability of the cardiovascular system to meet aerobic demands for certain activities. Patients unable to perform moderate activity such as walking 2–3 miles per hour or perform basic household chores are at an increased perioperative cardiac risk. Patients who exhibit no limitations or only slight limitations when they perform ordinary activities and who do not have symptoms such as angina or an anginal equivalent are considered low-risk for major surgical procedures, and likewise, suitable for sedation and analgesia.

For patients with a prior cardiac history, the presence of an old medical chart provides valuable documentation of hospitalizations, electrocardiograms, and diagnostic tests. Table 1 itemizes some of the more useful tests and their results.

One need not repeat tests if they have been done; if the patient's health has not changed, an EKG or other dignostic tests from even 2 years prior to the evaluation appears to be sufficient.

Pulmonary Abnormalities

Medications that produce sedation and analgesia affect pulmonary function by depressing the ventilatory response to both hypercarbia and hypoxia. Patients with pulmonary disease are at risk for periprocedural complications resulting from problems with ventilation and oxygenation. A preprocedure assessment that is able to identify patients at risk for pulmonary complications should focus on the following historical elements:

History of Respiratory Disease. Significant categories of pulmonary disease to ask of patients include chronic obstructive pulmonary disease (emphysema, chronic bronchitis), asthma, recent infection (viral, bacterial pneumonia), use of supplemental oxygen.

Chronic bronchitis is a clinical diagnosis characterized by a productive cough for consecutive months in 2 or more successive years. Emphysema results from destruction of alveolar units, leading to abnormal enlargement of airspaces distal to the terminal bronchioles. Smoking is the primary cause of both forms of chronic obstructive pulmonary disease (COPD). Sputum production and secretion mobilization are key issues for these patients, particularly during sedation when the patient's ventilatory responses are depressed. The use of postprocedural maneuvers such as postural drainage may help with sputum clearance. Patients may have problems lying flat due to respiratory problems. Patients in whom disease is severe enough to warrant supplemental oxygen at baseline should be supplied with the same level of oxygen throughout the procedure and during the recovery period to maintain oxygen saturations above 90%. The use of bronchodilator medications, including beta adrenergic agonists and corticosteroids, will aid in the pulmonary management and should be used until the time of the procedure and after the procedure if necessary. Finally, positioning patients with chronic obstructive lung disease if very important. Head-down or lateral positions can significantly compromise respiratory function and may not be tolerated by patients who have minimal respiratory reserve. If such positioning is warranted, patients may require endotracheal intubation and mechanical ventilation. Patients who have chronic obstructive airway disease should be as upright as possible during any procedure to optimize lung function.

The preprocedural evaluation of asthma follows the same guidelines as those for COPD. Since the airway tone is hyperreactive in asthmatic patients, procedures that take place in or around the airway may stimulate an asthmatic attack. Medications used to control airway tone (β-adrenergic agonist inhalers) and anti-inflammation medications (corticosteroids) can effectively control the symptoms of asthma. Elective procedures should be canceled if the patient has problems with asthma control.

Viral respiratory infections may lead to increased airway reactivity and airway obstruction. Bacterial infections should be treated with antibiotics and cleared prior to the procedure.

Description of Current Symptoms. An especially important symptom to document in detail is dyspnea, defined as an uncomfortable sensation of breathing. As in the case of angina, the degree of dyspnea can be accorded a grade or category, which correlates with postoperative survival. Because patients are required to maintain their own airway with spontaneous ventilation during sedation and analgesia, dyspnea on mild exertion or at rest should prompt further evaluation of the cause of dyspnea and the institution of appropriate treatment if possible. If evaluation reveals poor ventilatory reserve or predicts a need for postprocedure ventilatory support, outpatient sedation might not be a reasonable choice.

History of Smoking. Tobaccco consumption is measured in pack-years. Tobacco use results in higher pulmonary complications compared with non-smokers.

Body Habitus. Patients with spinal deformities (kyphoscoliosis) or obesity run a higher risk of developing atelectasis and hypoxemia during periods of ventilatory depression due to compression of lung volumes and a decrease in pulmonary compliance. They also tolerate positions, other than sitting upright, poorly. Even the supine position in morbidly obese patients can be associated with significant hypoxemia.

History of Cardiovascular Disease. Patients with chronic obstructive pulmonary disease also may have pulmonary hypertension and right heart failure. Symptoms and signs associated with these conditions should be sought, as patients who have significant pulmonary hypertension do not tolerate decreases in their blood pressure nor do they tolerate hypoxia or hypercapnia. Patients with sleep apnea and chronic airway obstruction (i.e., enlarged tonsils) also can have pulmonary hypertension and right heart failure.

Endocrine Abnormalities

Patients with diabetes require special evaluation and consideration for all procedures that require sedation. This is because of their multisystem disease as well as their medications, which result in hypoglycemia. Patients with diabetes, both type I and type II, have multiple end-organ problems due to long-standing uncontrolled blood glucose levels. All diabetics have an increased incidence of cardiac disease and may also have gastrointestinal disease, and are always at risk for increased rates of infection after procedures.

The preprocedure evaluation of diabetic patients requires a summary of their disease type and duration, documentation of their medical therapy, an assessment of end-organ involvement, and ultimately communication with the patient regarding management of blood glucose in the periprocedural period. The management goal of the diabetic patient during sedation and analgesia is to avoid wide swings in glycemic control, electrolyte abnormalities, and ketoacidosis.

Type I (insulin-dependent) diabetes mellitus is an autoimmune disorder resulting in destruction of the pancreatic islet cells that produce insulin. Onset of the disease occurs at a young age, and it is treated with insulin.

Type II (insulin-independent) diabetes mellitus, far more common than type I, is a disorder of resistance to the effects of insulin. Onset is usually in adulthood and it is often associated with obesity. Glucose levels can be controlled with dietary measures, oral hypoglycemic medications, and/or insulin.

End-Organ Complications of Diabetes

Diabetes results in atherosclerotic vascular disease and autonomic and peripheral neuropathies, which combine to affect many of the major organ systems and extremities.

Cardiovascular Complications. Coronary artery disease and myocardial ischemia is common among diabetics. Because of neuropathy, myocardial ischemia is often silent and goes unrecognized by the patient. A review of the old chart, with studies such as electrocardiograms, and a thorough cardiac history and physical examination should clarify the extent of the patient's cardiac disease. If the patient has not had an electrocardiogram within the previous year, it is reasonable to obtain one prior to an elective procedure involving sedation.

Pulmonary Complications. Autonomic neuropathy also may decrease the ventilatory drive in response to hypoxia and to medications that promote respiratory depression.

Gastrointestinal Complications. Gastroparesis, or delayed emptying of the gut, is a result of diabetic autonomic neuropathy. Because of the higher risk of full stomach in these patients, all diabetics should either receive aspiration prophylaxis, consisting of an H2-blocking medication, possibly a gut motility–promoting agent, and a non-particulate antacid or they should be considered for endotracheal intubation for airway protection. Periprocedural nausea and vomiting occurs as a result of gastroparesis and should be treated pre-emptively and aggressively to avoid aspiration.

Renal Complications. Diabetic nephropathy will be revealed in a urinalysis. Significant proteinuria may result in hypoalbuminemia with third-spacing. Peripheral edema, pulmonary effusion, and ascites all have respiratory implications for patients undergoing sedation and analgesia. Scheduling of a procedure may need to be coordinated with dialysis for patients with end-stage renal disease. Many of the drugs used in sedation or their metabolites are metabolized by the kidney. Morphine has a metabolite that is excreted by the kidneys and thus late respiratory depression can be seen in diabetes patients with renal failure who receive "normal" doses of morphine.

Extremities. Peripheral neuropathies and symptoms must be documented prior to positioning, as these patients are at higher risk for injury.

Periprocedural Glycemic Control. Blood glucose levels between 120 and 200 mg/dl have become the standard goal for maintaining control of electrolytes, fluid status, and acidosis. Patients should avoid solid foods after midnight prior to the procedure. Oral hypoglycemics should be held 24 hours prior to the procedure. Insulin should be held on the morning of the procedure. Ideally, glucose levels should be checked just prior to the procedure. Where possible, electrolytes should also be checked, including magnesium and phosphate.

Finally, diabetics often have visual impairment or are blind. If the patient cannot read, instructions need to be read to them and care must be taken to ensure that the patient has assistance after a procedure involving sedation.

Physical Examination

The physical examination for sedation and analgesia should focus on the airway, heart, lungs, and extremities. The neurologic status of the patient also deserves attention.

Vital Signs. Prior to the commencement of the procedure, blood pressure, heart rate, and oxygen saturation should be recorded as a baseline set of values. The patient's weight is important for calculating drug dosages. For patients with a history of cardiac or pulmonary disease, the respiratory rate at rest should be documented. Temperature should be noted, particularly in children. Febrile patients probably should not be considered for elective procedures involving sedation.

Airways. The airway exam should begin with noting the body habitus of the patient. Obesity, especially involving the face and neck, may lead to difficulties in spontaneous ventilation under sedation and analgesia. Other abnormalities to document include small mouth opening (3 finger breadths or less), loose or carious teeth, large tongue, and nonvisible uvula.

Neck. The thyromental distance should be measured (< 3 finger breadths may result in poor visualization of vocal cords). Observe cervical range of motion, especially neck extension and flexion. If the patient cannot move the head because of physical abnormalities or symptoms, this should be noted and means the endotracheal intubation of this patient could be difficult. Auscultate for carotid bruits. The presence of carotid bruits deserves further evaluation, since greater than 70% stenosis of the carotid artery is associated with adverse outcomes in noncardiac surgeries. Look for jugular venous distention as a sign of congestive heart failure.

Lungs. Auscultate for rales, rhonchi, inspiratory and expiratory wheezing. Observe use of accessory muscles during respiration.

Heart. Auscultate the precordium for a third heart sound, irregular rhythms, and murmurs. Tachycardia and bradycardia indicate a need for an electrocardiogram (unless previously identified).

Extremities. The presence of lower extremity peripheral edema requires further evaluation to rule out congestive heart failure, right-sided heart failure, deep venous thrombosis, and liver disease. Peripheral sensory or motor dysfunction should be documented. Diabetic patients with peripheral neuropathies are susceptible to nerve injury when improperly positioned.

Neurologic Status. Intact mental status and cognition are important to document prior to sedation and analgesia. The patient must be able to respond to verbal command during the procedure while under the influence of sedatives. Maintenance of a patent airway requires a functional gag reflex for protection.

Aspiration Risk

Sedation and analgesia are associated with a risk of aspiration, since the airway is not protected by an endotracheal tube and reflexes may be decreased by the medication. Recognizing which patients are at risk is the first step in the prevention of aspiration. Obesity, diabetes, pregnancy, difficult airway, recent meal, recent ethanol ingestion, bowel obstruction, and reflux disease are conditions associated with regurgitation and aspiration. Patients should receive clear instructions about undergoing an adequate fasting period prior to the procedure. All patients who appear to be at risk for aspiration should be considered for nonparticulate antacid, and if necessary, an H2-blocker to neutralize or decrease stomach acid production prior to the procedure.

Patient Considerations Affect the Choice of Medications Used for Sedation and Analgesia

In procedures that use sedation and analgesia, complications most often arise not from the procedure itself but rather from the patient's response to the sedative and analgesic medications. These adverse drug events include respiratory depression, hypoxia, and unwanted cardiovascular events.[3] When guided by an understanding of the pharmacology of sedatives and analgesics, the practitioner performing the preprocedure assessment can identify patients at high risk for complications, which in turn will influence intraprocedural management of the patient. While pharmacology is more thoroughly reviewed in other chapters, what follows is a discussion of the effect of patient assessment on the choice of the drugs used during outpatient procedures.

Adverse Reactions

The goal of sedation and analgesia is to provide comfort to the patient while keeping airway reflexes intact. Sedation prior to and during the procedure is used to reduce anxiety and allows the patient to tolerate minimal levels of discomfort. Analgesia, usually in the form of opioids, provides relief from pain of injection of local anesthetic and discomfort from nonincisional factors. When these two drugs are used in combination, there is an increased chance of significant respiratory depression in the form of decreased tidal volume and slowed respiratory rate, blunting of airway reflexes, respiratory obstruction, and depression of ventilatory responses to hypoxemia and hypercarbia.[1,2] In addition to the respiratory effects, sedatives and analgesics also exert depressant effects on the the cardiovascular system. A decrease in blood pressure and heart rate occurs to some degree after the administration of either the sedatives or the opioids. When sedatives and analgesics are used in combination, the magnitude and duration of these depressant effects can be additive or supra-additive (synergistic). Therefore, any time these drugs are used together and especially when they are used in combination in very fragile patients, there should be a significant decrease in the dosages of both classes of drugs.

Special care must be taken to adjust dosages when these drugs are used in the elderly or in patients with significant disease of the major organs. In contrast, patients with a history of substance abuse (tobacco, alcohol, intravenous drugs, etc.), chronic pain treated with opioids, or those who often ingest sedatives may require increased dosages for adequate sedation or analgesia.[5]

Benzodiazepines

The benzodiazepines are the most commonly used drugs for reducing preprocedure anxiety, and for providing intraprocedural sedation. Midazolam (Versed) is widely used because it has a rapid onset of action and profound sedative and amnestic effects. Because of its potency, the use of midazolam requires greater vigilance for unwanted side effects such as respiratory depression and excessive sedation.[7] Diazepam (Valium) also produces anxiolysis and amnesia, but has a significantly longer elimination half-life than midazolam and may result in delayed recovery.[6] Midazolam and diazepam are metabolized in the liver, and their activity is thus affected by such factors as age, liver disease, and drug interactions. Patient factors that require reduced dosages of benzodiazepines include advanced age, liver disease, and renal disease. In contrast, patients with a history of alcohol and tobacco use, or those who take benzodiazepines on a regular basis often require an increased dosage to reach an adequate effect.

Opioids

Opioids (fentanyl, alfentanil, remifentanil) provide effective analgesia for the pain and discomfort of procedures that are performed under conscious sedation. However, opioids also cause dose-dependent respiratory depression by decreasing central ventilatory drive, and their use must be carefully considered in patients with lung disease.[9] To minimize the risk of respiratory depression, dosages of opioids should be carefully titrated to effect, especially when used in conjunction with benzodiazepines.[2] Elderly patients are extremely sensitive to the therapeutic as well as to the side effects of opioids. Postprocedure nausea and vomiting increase with the use of opioids. Patient factors that increase the incidence of nausea and vomiting include young age, female gender, obesity, history of motion sickness, anxiety, and history of gastroparesis (i.e., associated with diabetes).

Propofol

Propofol is a sedative-hypnotic that is prepared in the form of an emulsion containing soybean oil, glycerol, egg protein, and an antibacterial agent. It is rapidly metabolized in the liver and excreted in the kidneys. As a result, hepatic disease will prolong the elimination of propofol. The popularity of propofol among anesthesiologists stems from its potency of effect, fast onset of action, and quick patient recovery. Propofol causes dose-dependent hypotension due to peripheral vasodilation and myocardial depression. Airway reflexes are depressed and apnea occurs even at "light" sedation doses. As with benzodiazepines and opioids, the cardiovascular and pulmonary effects of propofol are pronounced when used in elderly patients and in patients who have cardiac and pulmonary disease.

References

1.   Alexander CM, Gross JB: Sedative doses of midazolam depress hypoxic ventilatory responses in humans. Anesth Analg 67:377, 1988.
2.   Bailey PL, Pace NL, Ashburn MA, et al: Frequent hypoxemia and apnea after sedation with midazolam and fentanyl. Anesthesiology 73:826, 1990.
3.   Coplans MP, Curson I: Deaths associated with dentistry. Br Dent J 153:357, 1982.
4.   Klatsky AL: Cardiovascular effects of alcohol. Sci Am Med 2:28–37, 1995.
5.   Miller LG: Chronic benzodiazepine administration: From the patient to the gene. J Clin Pharmacol 31:492, 1991.

6. Mould DR, DeFeo TM, Reele S, et al: Simultaneous modeling of the pharmacokinetics and pharmacodynamics of midazolam and diazepam. Clin Pharmacol Ther 58:35, 1995.

7. Reves JG, Fragen RJ, Vinik H ret al: Midazolam: Pharmacology and uses. Anesthesiology 62:310, 1985.

8. Warner MA, Offerd KP, Warner ME, et al: Role of preoperative cessation of smoking and other factors in postoperative pulmonary complications: A blinded prospective study of coronary artery bypass patients. Mayo Clin Proc 64:609, 1989.

9. Weil JV, McCullough RE, Kline JS, et al: Diminished ventilatory response to hypoxia and hypercapnia after morphine in normal man. N Engl J Med 292:103, 1975.

4

Sedation in the Outpatient Setting

Ludwig H. Lin, M.D.

In the current health care environment, an increasing number of procedures in various specialties are being performed in same-day surgery facilities or in office-based settings. A number of these procedures performed by various specialists, including oral surgery, plastic surgery, ophthalmology, and otolaryngology, require some level of sedation. Using same-day, "come-and-go" models for such procedures is driven as much by economics as by patient satisfaction. In our competitive health care market, the savings gained from a decreased number of hospitalizations are relevant and essential for continued financial stability. At the same time, patients prefer to convalesce in the comfort of their own homes rather than in the unfamiliar, intimidating environment of a hospital. The increasing role of adequate sedation in the success of these procedures is also explained by the health care professional's recognition of the importance of patient comfort and satisfaction. For many of these procedures, the ability of the provider to offer sedation as part of the procedure lessens, for the patient, the anxiety associated with any medical procedure. Of course, in the case of the pediatric population, sedation is practically essential for certain procedures.

The intent of this chapter is to discuss some fundamental principles a nonanesthesiologist should consider when designing sedation protocols for procedures in the outpatient setting. The advantages and disadvantages of the use of various sedation agents in the ambulatory setting are discussed. In addition to providing guidelines with regard to the equipment and medications one should have in the office as part of the set-up for providing sedation, medical conditions that should not be treated on an outpatient basis are discussed.

Physical Setup

There are regulations on the city, state, and federal levels as well as by various specialty organizations describing the essential safety features required for the practice of outpatient sedation. The Joint Commission on Accreditation of Healthcare Organizations (JCAHO) has established guidelines from which many hospitals have adapted their ambulatory surgery and office-based sedation guidelines. The Accreditation Association for Ambulatory Health Care (AAAHC), an organization that inspects and accredits office-based health care, also has published guidelines.[1,6,11,13,24,26]

In terms of the physical layout, the procedure room has to be separated from the recovery area. This is also an efficient set-up, as recovering patients are removed from the operating area so that patient flow can continue. Furthermore, this is essential to ensure patient privacy and safety. Patients undergoing procedures should not be sharing the space with recovering patients. Also, there needs to be dedicated personnel whose sole responsibility is to monitor recovering patients.

The areas should all be well lit, with clear signs indicating the emergency exits. The rooms and the hallways need to have space free of equipment so that patients, their gurneys, and health care personnel can maneuver easily. Emergency power needs to be available to power the resuscitation equipment. The various pieces of equipment need to be grounded and electrically isolated from each other to prevent current induction and unintended electric shocks.

Personnel needs to be trained in the skills necessary for providing sedation, as well as handling the possible side effects of sedation. They need to be able to take standard vital signs, to be able to administer sedative-hypnotics and opiates safely (i.e., possess an understanding of the pharmacology and possible interactions involved with the administration of such agents), and to recognize potentially life-threatening situations (such as hypotension, respiratory depression, apnea, and possible respiratory collapse).

All personnel responsible for patient care needs to be familiar with advanced cardiac life support (ACLS) and airway equipment. The ACLS training needs to be repeated every 2 years. Similar to the training required to use medical equipment, it is important to document that refresher courses or in-service training opportunities are available to personnel and when they have taken these courses.

Equipment for monitoring a patient's vital signs, maintaining adequate oxygenation, and performing emergent resuscitation should be present at all times. At the same time, a clearly stated schedule of maintainance and quality control of such equipment should be established to assure proper functioning of equipment.

Vital signs are monitored at periodic intervals; the suggested frequency of monitoring for sedation is every 15 minutes. The existence of automated blood pressure measuring devices (Dyna-map), continuous percutaneous oxygen saturation monitoring devices, and even simple capnography devices have made the monitoring of deeply sedated patients easier and safer.

Adequate oxygenation can be monitored by continuous percutaneous oxygen saturation devices. Supplemental oxygen has to be available, either as a built-in wall source or as portable oxygen cylinders. Nasal cannulae, face masks, and positive-pressure ventilation devices (the self-inflating Ambu-Bag and the Jackson-Rees circuit, tight-sealing face masks) should be available to deliver various concentrations of oxygen to the patients. For the situation in which a patient needs to be resuscitated with positive-pressure ventilation, an anesthesia mask with an inflatable cuff should be available to provide for a tight seal on the patient's face. Different sizes of masks for patients ranging from neonates to large adults should be available if different age groups are treated.

To deal with upper airway obstruction, devices such as nasal airways and oral airways of various sizes should be available. However, endotracheal intubation should only be attempted by someone skilled in this procedure (i.e., an anesthesiologist or others trained in advanced airway management, such as oral surgeons or dentists certified in anesthesia). Nevertheless, at least one of the attending personnel should be proficient in mask ventilation so that ventilation can be maintained until help arrives or a patient is transferred to a hospital setting.

The ability to suction the patient emergently during an episode of regurgitation is essential. A vacuum source, Yankauer suction device, and suction tubing need to be available and in the vicinity of the patient. Emergency equipment, such as a transcutaneous pacer/defibrillator or an automated defibrillator device (AED), needs to be on standby as well.

Other necessary equipment includes syringes, needles or needleless injection port systems, intravenous (IV) tubing, and IV fluids. The standard maintenance IV fluids are the crystalloid solutions of either normal saline (0.9% sodium chloride) or balanced salt solutions (lactated Ringer, Plasma-Lyte). Intravenous access kits (IV catheters, sterile dressings) are now designed to minimize the risk of needlestick injuries to the health care professionals; their use is relatively complicated and may necessitate an initial training session for the clinic personnel.

Patient Assessment and Consent

Before a patient undergoes sedation and a procedure, a history and physical examination should be performed and documented in the patient's medical record. This assessment needs to document that the patient is medically fit and can withstand the procedure as well as the sedation.

A consent form should be signed by all patients stating that they understand the risks and benefits of the procedure as well as the sedation, that they are aware of alternatives to the current proposed plan, and that they are willing to proceed. For minors, the consent has to be signed by the parents or guardians.

Contraindications to Undergoing Sedation

Certain patients with severe underlying medical problems should not under-go an office-based procedure, but might be able to have the same procedure done when advanced airway skills and cardiopulmonary resuscitation are available (i.e., anesthesiologist or other trained personnel). Patients with dementia may not be able to follow any commands and may react to sedation with paradoxical disin-hibition and agitation. Patients with congestive heart failure, cardiomyopathy or other cardiopulmonary disease may not be able to lie down and thus would be poor candidates for sedation. The situation is similar for patients with severe pul-monary diseases such as chronic obstructive pulmonary disease (COPD). Patients who have CO_2 retention and thus, by definition, have abnormal respiratory drives, may respond to sedative agents with marked respiratory depression. Patients with severe pulmonary hypertension, i.e., systolic pulmonary arterial pressures above 40 mmHg, can have hyperreactive pulmonary vasculature that constricts in response to hypoxia, hypercarbia, pain, or agitation. Therefore, out-patient sedation may be dangerous for these patients as it could precipitate increased pulmonary pressures and thus cause right-heart failure. Patients with severe symptoms of reflux or known anatomic diseases predisposing to reflux, such as hiatal hernias, esophageal strictures, and achalasia, are at increased risk for regurgitation and aspiration. In these patients, the removal of their protective air-way reflexes by deep sedation might precipitate regurgitation and aspiration.

NPO Status

The NPO status is controversial, because maintaining strict "nothing by mouth past midnight" is difficult for most patients. However, because of the potential loss of protective airway reflexes during sedation, even if the original intent is to start with light, "conscious" sedation, anesthesiologists strictly enforce the rule of 8 hours of NPO. For patients on chronic antihypertensive or antiang-inal therapy it has become the standard of care to continue these medications, as discontinuing the medications may lead to hypertension and/or angina. Therefore, the patients are permitted to ingest their medications with a sip of water as early as possible prior to the onset of the procedure and the administra-tion of sedation.

In the pediatric population (see Chapter 7), children younger than 2 need to stop intake of solid food and full liquids 6 hours prior to the procedure, but may take clear liquids up to 2 hours prior to the procedure. Children ages 2–4 can take clear liquids up to 4 hours prior to the procedure. Children older than 6 should follow the adult guidelines. Clear liquids include water, black coffee, breast milk, cranberry and apple juice, and non-particulate grape juice.[11,13,19,21,24]

Pregnancy

Women past the first trimester of pregnancy should be considered as having a full stomach, and are at increased risk for regurgitation and aspiration. The risks versus benefits of conducting a sedated procedure in this population need to be carefully considered. When conducting a procedure on women in the last trimester of pregnancy, the issue of fetal well-being becomes relevant, because a fetus in the 28th week of gestation is viable when delivered prematurely. Therefore, if a woman in such an advanced stage of pregnancy is to be sedated, fetal monitoring should be done. This is probably best done in a hospital setting.

Medications

A variety of agents are used to achieve sedation. The main classes of medications are discussed, along with their major characteristics that may cause untoward consequences.

Sedative/Hypnotics

Sedative/hypnotic agents are drugs that decrease a person's level of alertness, provide for anxiolysis, and perhaps even supply amnesia. The major classes of sedative/hypnotics include barbiturates, benzodiazepines, and propofol.

The barbiturates and benzodiazepines share some common side effects, including somnolence. Cross-tolerance in patients who abuse substances such as ethanol occurs, although the cross-tolerance does not seem to be equally evident for all of the sedative-hypnotic effects. For example, the lethal dose ranges are not affected, while the doses required for adequate sedation and anxiolysis are.

Benzodiazepines

Benzodiazepines act on the GABA receptors of the central nervous system. The current theory is the GABA receptor, a chloride anion channel protein, has an inhibitory effect on the central nervous system when stimulated. It is a complex of three receptor molecules binding to GABA, barbiturates, and benzodiazepines. The binding of benzodiazepines prolongs and increases the effects of GABA activation. At high concentrations, benzodiazepines may have GABA-mimetic effects.[16]

Some commonly used benzodiazepines include lorazepam (Ativan), diazepam (Valium), midazolam (Versed), temazepam (Restoril), alprazolam (Xanax), and clonazepam (Klonopin). They provide sedation and anxiolysis; hypnosis, or induction of sleep, is also caused by these drugs. These drugs can also cause amnesia. They are sometimes also used as muscle relaxants. The onset time ranges from a few minutes for midazolam to 15–30 minutes for lorazepam and diazepam.[20] The duration of action varies widely, from 2–4 hours for midazolam, to 50–150 hours for diazepam. For office-based procedures, midazolam and lorazepam are the most useful choices; they offer reasonably short onset times, and allow patients to recover within 2–3 hours, so that the patients can return home safely.

All of the benzodiazepines are metabolized by the liver. Most of the members have active metabolites, which are cleared by further hepatic metabolism or renal excretion. In patients with hepatic dysfunction, the delayed metabolism of both the parent compound as well as its metabolites can cause vastly prolonged and exaggerated drug effects. Lorazepam, flurazepam, and temazepam are the three benzodiazepines that are metabolized to inactive metabolites.[16] Patients who have cirrhosis can therefore be oversedated with standard doses of benzodiazepines. Benzodiazepines should be avoided in patients who have a history consistent with severe hepatic failure, such as hepatic encephalopathy, baseline coagulopathy, or recurrent ascites, since those are markers of decreased hepatic synthetic function.

Benzodiazepines also are known to cause paradoxical effects, particularly in the elderly population. In the elderly, benzodiazepines have been reported to cause disinhibition and agitated behavior. This disinhibition may manifest as an inability to follow intraprocedural commands to remain still or quiet, which may adversely affect the procedure. Furthermore, there have been data suggesting that benzodiazepine administration is associated with prolonged cognitive problems in elderly patients.

In uncooperative children, an oral or subcutaneous dose of benzodiazepines is often administered. Those dosing routes need a longer time of onset and require larger quantities of drugs to achieve an effect. Using benzodiazepines by these routes can cause a prolonged duration of action due to the larger doses administered, as well as because a depot of medications is formed that results in gradual systemic absorption.

When administered alone, benzodiazepines do not depress the respiratory center in the central nervous system. However, in select populations, they can cause respiratory problems. Patients who have a predilection for upper airway obstruction may be so precarious that any muscle relaxation, e.g., resulting from the use of benzodiazepines, can result in airway obstruction and subsequent respiratory compromise. For example, patients with pickwickian syndrome (central hypoventilation syndrome), extreme obesity, sleep apnea, or known previous episodes of upper airway obstruction are poor candidates for sedation with benzodiazepines. Furthermore, benzodiazepines have a synergistic depressant effect on respiratory drive when coadministered with opiates or barbiturates. In situations when various classes of medications are used concomitantly, the patient's respiratory status should be carefully monitored.

Barbiturates

Barbiturates are used in the same fashion as benzodiazepines. In small doses, they offer sedative-hypnotic properties. However, in larger doses they produce obtundation and can cause general anesthesia. They also have the potential for lethal complications, including respiratory depression, apnea, and cardiovascular collapse.

Methohexital, sodium thiopental, pentobarbital, and phenobarbital are some barbiturates used as agents for sedation. Phenobarbital is a long-acting barbiturate used as an antiseizure medication. Methohexital has a moderately long-elimination half-life, but has a rapid onset and a rapid clearance of sedative effects, because of its strong lipophilicity and large volume of distribution. Used sparingly, i.e., not in a repeated dosing regimen where it can accumulate in the tissues and cause prolonged sedative effects, methohexital can be used effectively in the outpatient setting.

Methohexital can be administered via intravenous or rectal routes, and can be given as either intravenous/rectal boluses or as an intravenous infusion. Again, like the benzodiazepines, the clearance rates of this drug are decreased in patients with hepatic dysfunction. Interestingly, prolonged use of barbiturates, as well the use of some other medications like phenytoin, leads to an upregulation of the hepatic clearance enzymes and is associated with a shortened duration of action.

Like the benzodiazepines, barbiturates also have muscle relaxation effects. Unlike the benzodiazepines, however, at higher dosages the barbiturates cause direct respiratory depression. This leads to hypoventilation and apnea. Barbiturates also cause significant myocardial depression and can reduce the systemic vascular resistance. Thus, the administration of barbiturates is associated with lowered cardiac outputs and decreased blood pressures. These cardiovascular effects can be exaggerated in patients whose cardiovascular system is already compromised, such as patients who are dehydrated or patients who have cardiac dysfunction.

Propofol

Propofol is similar to benzodiazepines and barbiturates in that it acts as a sedative/hypnotic; it is more like barbiturates than benzodiazepines in that it serves as a sedative/amnesiac agent at lower doses, and achieves general anesthesia at higher doses. It has the same ability as the barbiturates to produce respiratory depression and hemodynamic instability. The advantage of propofol, which is the only drug in its class, is that it is cleared very efficiently by the body. Although it is metabolized partly by the liver, propofol can be cleared even in patients who have no hepatic function, such as patients during the anhepatic phase of a liver transplant surgery, and thus there must be nonspecific metabolism of this drug in the plasma. The advantage of this nonspecific metabolic pathway is that prolonged administration of propofol does not lead to its accumulation in peripheral tissues, and thus does not lead to prolonged sedation. It has a rapid onset time (within seconds) and a rapid offset time (within 10–15 minutes of the cessation of an infusion). Propofol is used as a continuous intravenous infusion. It is suspended as an emulsification in preservative-laden lipids. It can cause pain when it is injected; the pain is caused by irritation of the venous endothelium. Furthermore, there are possible allergic reactions that should be noted. The emulsion will cause an allergic reaction in people allergic to either soy proteins or egg-white proteins, and the preservatives (EDTA or sulfa compounds) also are known allergens.

Propofol is a powerful sedative/hypnotic, and should be used only in situations where a person who is trained in advanced airway management is available. At the usual sedation doses of 25–75 µg/kg/min, significant respiratory depression should not occur. However, various comorbid conditions in a particular patient may cause respiratory distress at these usually safe doses. These conditions include obesity, a propensity for upper airway obstruction, the administration of other sedation agents, or advanced age. Therefore, when administering propofol, there is always the possibility that a patient may require aggressive airway management.

Ketamine

Ketamine may be a useful agent in the outpatient setting. It is a derivative of phencyclidine (PCP), and produces "dissociative anesthesia," unlinking the limbic system from the rest of the brain. It produces profound analgesia, amnesia, and catatonia, while maintaining respiratory drive and upper airway musculature tone. It is its ability to maintain the respiratory function that makes it a good agent for outpatient sedation.[18] Compared to the other agents mentioned above, for an equal level of analgesia and amnesia, ketamine is the least likely compound to cause respiratory compromise. It also is a sympathomimetic, meaning that it tends to maintain or even increase the patient's blood pressure rather than produce hypotension. It also is short-acting and clears within 20–30 minutes.

On the other hand, ketamine does have some undesirable side effects. It has sialogogic activity, producing increased oropharyngeal secretions, and can increase cerebral blood flow, cerebral oxygen consumption, and intracranial pressure. Because of its effects on the limbic system, it can cause hallucinations or dysphoric dreams. To prevent these problems, ketamine is often given in conjunction with a short-acting benzodiazepine that counters the incidence of hallucinations.[16]

Opioids

The elegant method of sedating a patient during a procedure requires some thought as to the reasons for the sedation—is the patient anxious regarding the procedure, thus requiring anxiolysis? Does the patient require a level of hypnosis to make him/her a little less arousable and thus make the procedure technically easier? Or, rather, is the procedure somewhat painful, thus necessitating the use of both topical anesthesia as well as systemic analgesia? If the last option is correct, a short-acting opioid should be added to the sedation regimen. However, when used in combination, all sedative agents tend to be additive or even synergistic in the production of respiratory depression. Therefore, opioids should be administered very carefully when given in combination with other agents, such as benzodiazepines or barbiturates.

Several different synthetic opioids are marketed for use in short, office-based procedures. The most frequently used compounds include: (1) the rapid-onset, short-acting agents such as alfentanil; (2) the rapid-onset, medium-duration agents such as sufentanil and fentanyl; (3) the medium-onset, medium-duration agents like morphine sulfate and hydromorphone; and (4) the ultrashort-acting compounds like remifentanil. Other agents, such as demerol, are also in use. Finally, partial agonist/antagonists of opioids, such as nalbuphine (Nubain) and butorphanol (Stadol), also are used.[16,26]

Opioids all work on opioid receptors, present in the brain and the spinal cord, as well as in the peripheral nerves. Different theories currently are attempting to explain the function of the utility of various receptors present at different regions of the nervous system. There are multiple receptor subtypes that produce slightly different effects when stimulated by the binding of an opioid compound.

For office-based procedures, the goals of opioid administration should be to produce a mild degree of analgesia as well as a mildly decreased level of consciousness. Also, opioids that have a short-duration of action should be administered, so the patient is not at risk of having respiratory depression at home. Usually, agents are administered that have a rapid onset of action, meaning that the analgesic effects occur rapidly, enhancing patient satisfaction. Once the desired level of analgesia and sedation has been obtained, the medium duration of effect of such opioids means that patients will recover in time to be discharged home, yet they will not have such complete resolution of the analgesic effects that they are immediately in pain following the procedure.

Fentanyl and sufentanil both have a rapid onset of action. Sufentanil is about five times more potent than fentanyl, which is in turn 100 times more potent than morphine sulfate. Fentanyl seems to be the opioid agent used in many outpatient sedation centers. Fentanyl actually has a slightly longer half-life than morphine—3.1 hours vs. 2.2 hours.[12] However, because of its higher lipophilicity, it has a shorter onset of action and is rapidly redistributed from the plasma into various tissue compartments. Therefore, the plasma level rapidly drops following the initial bolus, and its "context-sensitive" duration of action is shorter than that of morphine. These are the characteristics that endear fentanyl to an office-based practitioner.

With repeat dosing of either sufentanil (> 2 µg/kg) or fentanyl (> 5 µg/kg), the drugs will accumulate and cause prolonged effects. Remifentanil and alfentanil, while used by anesthesiologists, are probably too short-acting to be useful to nonanesthesiologists. Also, they can be associated with significant muscle rigidity that can preclude ventilation.

Morphine can be used in outpatient sedation settings. Its onset of action is slower, in the range of 10–15 minutes. However, its prolonged action provides for a long period of analgesia, which may be desirable in procedures associated with postprocedure pain.

Opioids are metabolized by the liver. In patients with hepatic dysfunction, their clearance may be compromised, and their effect on respiratory drive can be significantly prolonged. In patients with renal failure, the clearance of the metabolites of morphine (morphine-3-glucuronide and morphine-6-glucuronide) and of meperidine (normeperidine) is delayed, and they can accumulate and cause seizures (normeperidine) or prolonged respiratory depression (morphine-6-glucuronide).[20]

Partial agonist/antagonists, like nalbuphine and butorphanol, are used in outpatient settings because their partial antagonist properties supposedly prevent respiratory depression. Furthermore, recently women have been shown to respond to the analgesic effects of the kappa opioid agents (nalbuphine) to a greater degree than men, and this may be a useful characteristic to exploit in outpatient sedation settings.[12]

For improved analgesic effects, one can also administer the over-the-counter medications, including acetaminophen or one of the nonsteroidal anti-inflammatory drugs (NSAIDs), such as ibuprofen. These drugs have to be administered prior to the procedure, because the oral route of administration requires a longer time for onset of action. A method to achieve optimal results is to instruct the patient to ingest either acetaminophen or an NSAID on the morning of the procedure with a sip of water, provided that the patient does not have any contraindications to taking these drugs. By the time the patient is undergoing the procedure, these drugs will have produced a satisfactory plasma level, which should help to decrease the need for opiate analgesia. These compounds are useful because they do not cause an altered mental status nor do they have the respiratory obstruction/depressive effects of other analgesics. Acetaminophen has hepatic and renal effects, and should not be administered to patients who have hepatic dysfunction or consume alcohol. Furthermore, the daily dose of acetaminophen should not exceed 3 g. NSAIDs can cause gastrointestinal hemorrhage as well as renal problems, particularly in hypovolemic patients.[15]

There are other medications that are nonsedative hypnotics in that their primary effect is not sedation, but they do cause sedation or drowsiness as a side effect, and thus can be used as adjunctive agents. Antihistamines, such as diphenhydramine, phenothiazines like prochlorperazine (compazine), and butyrophenones—haloperidol (Haldol) and droperidol—are useful as adjunct sedatives. These agents have antimuscarinic effects that cause dry mouth. The butyrophenones also can have extrapyramidal effects and may even cause akathisia or the neuroleptic malignant syndrome.[16,20]

Achieving Desired Level of Sedation

Patient undergoing conscious sedation have an altered mood and a slightly sedated level of consciousness. They are awake and can cooperate with verbal commands. They have intact airway protective reflexes and a normal respiratory pattern. Because of the low doses of medications that are given for this level of sedation, these patients tend to have stable vital signs, but also do not have a lot of analgesia. Therefore, the procedure does not require anesthesia or only requires local anesthesia. The kind of agents recommended for these situations should be rapidly acting with a short duration of action. Benadryl or lorazepam may be useful as adjunctive therapies, although their duration of action is longer. Amnesia may or may not result from conscious sedation.

Recovery after Sedation

After the end of the procedure, a patient who has undergone sedation needs to have continued monitoring during the recovery phase. Supplemental oxygen should be administered until the patients reach their baseline oxygen saturation (can be on supplemental oxygen) or they maintain a saturation of greater than 95% on room air. Furthermore, the patient's vital signs should be monitored at 15-minute intervals until the patient is awake, alert, and meets discharge criteria.[24]

Commonly, recovery from sedation is separated into three stages. In the early recovery, patients awaken from sedation. In intermediate recovery, they regain full psychomotor function and resume physical activity, such as ambulation and consumption of fluids. In late recovery, which occurs over the next few days, patients regain full psychological and physical recovery.[9] Mirroring the first two stages of recovery, the organization of the recovery area can be separated into patients in phase I, where the patient recovers consciousness, and phase II, where the patient regains and demonstrates to the staff the ability to resume the activities of daily living.

TABLE 1. Discharge Scoring Systems

Aldrete Scoring System		PADSS	
Activity		*Vital Signs*	
Can move voluntarily or on command		Within 20% of preoperative value	2
4 extremities	2	20–40% of preoperative value	1
2 extremities	1	40% of preoperative value	0
0 extremities	0		
Respiration		*Ambulation and Mental Status*	
Can deep-breathe and cough freely	2	Oriented x 3 *and* steady gait	2
Dyspnea, shallow or limited breathing	1	Oriented x 3 *or* steady gait	1
Apneic	0	Neither	0
Circulation		*Pain, nausea, vomiting*	
Preoperative BP (mmHg)		Minimal	2
BP ± 20 mmHg of baseline	2	Moderate	1
BP ± 20–50 mmHg of baseline	1	Severe	0
BP ± 50 mmHg of baseline	0		
Consciousness		*Surgical Bleeding*	
Fully awake	2	Minimal	2
Arousable on calling	1	Moderate	1
Not responding	0	Severe	0
Color		*Intake and Output*	
Normal	2	Has had PO fluids *and* voided	2
Pale, dusky, blotchy	1	Has had PO fluid *or* voided	1
Cyanotic	0	Neither	0
Score of 10: ready for discharge		**Score ≥ 9: ready for discharge**	

Evaluating a patient for discharge involves striking a balance between patient convenience, minimizing the recovery time, and increasing the risk of having a patient return for post-sedation complications. Phase I and phase II recovery can be conveniently evaluated with the Aldrete Scoring System, the PADS system, or the Wetchler Guidelines.[2,3,5,7–10,14,17] In the latter, which use a set of clinical guidelines, a patient is monitored for stable vital signs, the ability to swallow and cough, the ability to walk, minimal nausea, vomiting, or dizziness, and the absence of respiratory distress.[27] The patient also needs to be alert and oriented. Once the patients meet the chosen criteria, they can be successfully discharged. These clinical parameters are vague, and can be made more rigorous by the application of the Aldrete Scoring System[2,3] or the Post-Anaesthesia Discharge Scoring System (PADSS),[10] which score the patient's vital signs and psychomotor skills both at baseline and after recovery (Table 1). If the patient's score after recovery indicates a return to baseline function, the patient is ready for discharge.[9]

Traditionally, discharge is not approved for patients who cannot tolerate oral intake of fluids, or who cannot void. Recently, a shift in this paradigm has occurred with the publication of studies that demonstrate that 20% of patients can be discharged without meeting the criteria of tolerating oral intake (i.e., earlier in their recovery) without necessitating a return admission. Additionally, the rate of nausea and emesis, as well as prolongation of stay, is increased in the pediatric population when they are required to take oral fluids. Therefore, it seems reasonable to not persist in requiring that patients tolerate oral intake before they go home.[22,23,25]

The issue of the ability to void is also a subject to reassessment. The rate of postoperative urinary retention is low, even in the pediatric and elderly male population. The more recent philosophy is that patients do not necessarily have to void before going home, with the understanding that they may need to return to a hospital if they are unable to void at home following discharge.

Certain activities of daily living need to be curtailed immediately postprocedure. While patients are able to resume all activities at home, they should not drive or resume high-risk work activities immediately after discharge. For sedation procedures lasting less than 2 hours, patients should be able to resume driving or other high-risk activities after 24 hours. If the sedation lasts longer than 2 hours, some have suggested that patients should refrain from driving for 48 hours.[18] However, this probably is not followed universally.

Discharge instructions should be given to the patient, not only verbally, but also in a printed or written format. This is necessary not only for documentation purposes, but also because patients often continue to have antegrade amnesia in the immediate recovery period due to the sedative-hypnotic agents received during the procedure, and they may forget verbal instructions.

An agreement with a hospital should be in place so that, if a patient does have prolonged sedation postprocedure or has other complications from either the procedure itself or from the sedation, the patient can be evaluated or given other care.[26]

Conclusion

Sedation is administered frequently and safely in many different outpatient settings, and the development of numerous fast-onset, rapid-offset agents has allowed more satisfactory sedation conditions for patients. However, outpatient sedation is associated with certain risks, and the practitioner needs to: (1) be aware of them; (2) deny outpatient sedation to certain patients; and (3) be prepared for complications in a well-planned manner. With a well-planned physical setup, satisfactory monitoring equipment, and a full complement of emergency equipment, a practitioner can administer sedation safely and without complications.

References

1. Accreditation Association for Ambulatory Health Care: AAAHC Standards. Wilmette, IL, Accreditation Association for Ambulatory Health Care.
2. Aldrete JA: Modifications to the postanesthesia score for use in ambulatory surgery. J Perianesth Nurs 13:148–155, 1998.
3. Aldrete J, Kroulik D: A postanesthetic recovery score. Anesth Analg 49:924–934, 1970.
4. Barash P, Cullen B, Stoelting R (eds): Clinical Anesthesia, 2nd ed. Philadelphia, J.B. Lippincott, 1992.
5. Baskett P, Vickers M: Driving after anaesthetics. BMJ 1:686–687, 1979.
6. CAMF Hospitals: The Official Handbook, 1998.
7. Chung F: Return to daily living function after outpatient anesthesia. Anesth Analg 78:S62, 1994.
8. Chung F: Recovery pattern and home-readiness after ambulatory surgery. Anesth Analg 80:896–902, 1995.
9. Chung F, Chan VW, Ong D: A post-anesthetic discharge scoring system for home readiness after ambulatory surgery. J Clin Anesth 7:500–506, 1995.
10. Chung F, Ong D, Seyone C: PADSS: A discriminative discharge index for ambulatory surgery. Anesthesiology 75:A1105, 1991.
11. Feldscot A: The new regulations on conscious sedation. N Y State Dent J 55:8–10, 1989.
12. Gear RW, Miaskowski C, Gordon NC, et al: Kappa-opioids produce significantly greater analgesia in women than in men. Nature Med 2:1248–1250, 1996.
13. Hall S: Ambulatory anesthesia outside the operating room. In Twersky RS (ed): The Ambulatory Anesthesia Handbook. St. Louis, Mosby, 1995, pp 361–398.
14. Herbert M, Healy E, Bourke J: Profile of recovery after general anesthesia. BMJ 286:1539–1542, 1983.
15. Karnik J, Chertow G: Analgesic-related renal disease: Causes, patients at risk, management. J Crit Illness 15:49–58, 2000.
16. Katzung B (ed): Basic and Clinical Pharmacology, 4th ed. Stamford, CT, Appleton & Lange, 1989.
17. Korttila K: Recovery and driving after brief anaesthesia. Anaesthetist 30:377–382, 1982.
18. Kohrs R, Durieux ME: Ketamine: Teaching an old drug new tricks. Anesth Analg 87:1186–1193, 1998.
19. Milford MA, Paluch TA: Ambulatory laparoscopic fundoplication. Surg Endosc 11:1150–1152, 1997.
20. Morgan G, Mikhail M (eds): Clinical Anesthesiology, 2nd ed. Stamford, CT, Appleton & Lange, 1996.
21. Ouellette RG: Controversial issues in outpatient anesthesia: Adult and pediatric. CRNA 10:2–5, 1999.
22. Patterson P: Discharge criteria: Are they keeping up with practices? OR Manager 15:1, 17, 19 passim, 1999.
23. Schreiner M, Nicolson SC, Martin T, Whitney L: Should children drink before discharge from day surgery? Anesthesiology 76:528–533, 1992.
24. SP Services: Conscious Sedation Guidelines. San Francisco, CA, San Francisco General Hospital, 1999.
25. SP Services: Discharge of adult and pediatric ambulatory surgery patients based upon discharge criteria. San Francisco, CA, San Francisco General Hospital, 1999.
26. Twersky RS (ed): The Ambulatory Anesthesia Handbook. St. Louis, Mosby, 1995.
27. Wetchler B: Problem solving in the postanesthesia care unit. In Wetchler B (ed): Anesthesia for Ambulatory Surgery. Philadelphia, J.B. Lippincott, 1990, pp 375–436.

5

Sedation in the Intensive Care Unit

Richard H. Savel, M.D.

Alhough potentially life-saving, the intensive care unit (ICU) experience often can be a psychologically stressful and physically painful one. Clinicians working in the ICU setting must be able to rapidly and accurately assess pain, agitation and anxiety, as well as deliver appropriate analgesia and anxiolytics. Sedation in the ICU poses unique challenges: patients often have systemic illness and multiple organ failure, are frequently hemodynamically unstable and may be sedated on the order of days to weeks rather than minutes to hours as in other settings. Given these complexities, this chapter provides an overview of the current therapeutic options available to the critical care clinician so that an optimal level of consciousness and pain relief may be attained. Specifically, it addresses the relevant pharmacodynamic and pharmacokinetic issues with regards to sedative drugs in order to assist the clinician in choosing the best therapy for their patients. Although pain control and sedation are somewhat inextricably linked, this chapter focuses primarily on sedation, defined as the provision of analgesia and meeting the anxiolytic, hypnotic, and amnestic needs of the patient.[24] Also discussed are some of the controversies in ICU sedation, such as the role of protocols in the ICU, and whether daily awakenings are beneficial to patients. The goals of this chapter are to: (1) provide the ICU health care provider with an improved understanding of the adverse effects of uncontrolled pain and anxiety in the ICU; (2) recommend a combination of therapies that alleviate pain and anxiety in the ICU that is specific to both a patient's hemodynamic status and the likely duration of sedation; (3) demonstrate accurate assessment of a patient's response anxiolytic/analgesic therapy; and (4) emphasize greater awareness of some of the current controversies in critical care sedation.

The ICU: A Source of Pain, Confusion, and Anxiety

Pain and anxiety are unfortunate side effects of the various procedures performed in a modern ICU. In addition to the obvious unpleasant sensory input, under- or untreated pain has adverse consequences such as hypercoagulability and immunosuppression. Pain can contribute to a stress response, produced by stimulation of the peripheral, central, and autonomic nervous system as well as release of humoral factors such as kinins, leukotrienes, and prostaglandins. This mediator release can lead to increases in cardiac morbidity as well. Pain and anxiety also affect the pulmonary system, with a restrictive pattern, such as decreased vital and inspiratory capacities, most often being seen.[6]

From a physiologic standpoint, undertreatment of pain and anxiety can lead to hypertension, tachycardia, and ventilator dyssynchrony. Oversedation, in contradistinction, runs the risk of respiratory depression, hypotension, bradycardia, adynamic ileus, renal failure, venous stasis, and immunosuppression. Despite the best efforts of critical care clinicians to strike a balance between anxiety and complete unresponsiveness, the psychological ramifications of an ICU stay remain significant. One survey-based study revealed that 40% of critically ill patients discharged from an ICU recall having pain and 55% reported anxiety during their stay.[17] In another study, up to 50% described mechanical ventilation as unpleasant and stressful, leading to feelings of helplessness, fear, agony, and panic.[4]

Pain and Sedation Scales

A pain-free state must be obtained in the ICU patient prior to therapeutic intervention with sedating drugs, as pain itself can exacerbate anxiety and it is medically suboptimal to sedate a patient who may be in pain. It cannot be overemphasized that although sedation can be a side effect of opioids, benzodiazepines and other sedative agents are not analgesics per se and should not be used as such. As an initial step, the patient must be evaluated for any pain he or she may be suffering. Although a variety of methods are used to evaluate pain, rating scales are most commonly used. Of those, the visual analog scale (VAS) is the most widely accepted and, despite its apparent simplicity, has a great degree of validity and inter-observer reproducibility.[9] The most commonly used is a horizontal scale ranging from "no pain" to "the most pain I have ever had." Given that it is linear, the VAS is unable to convey the subtle multifactorial nuances of pain sensation. Other tests, such as the McGill Pain Questionnarie, have been designed to transmit such information. Its requirement for minimal interactivity, however, gives the VAS a distinct advantage in the ICU. Attempts have been made to correlate facial expressions and hemodynamic parameters such as tachycardia and hypertension with pain; however, these factors generally are too nonspecific to be of real value in assessing ICU pain.

Once the pain status of the patient has been assessed and appropriate analgesia has been delivered, the patient must be evaluated for level of sedation. The

TABLE 1. Ramsay Scale for Evaluating Level of Sedation in Critically Ill Patients

Level		Response
Awake levels	1	Patient anxious and agitated or restless or both
	2	Patient cooperative, oriented, and tranquil
	3	Patient responds to commands only
Asleep levels	4	Brisk response to a light glabellar tap or loud auditory stimulus
	5	Sluggish response to a light glabellar tap or loud auditory stimulus
	6	No response to a light glabellar tap or loud auditory stimulus

primary measure of sedation in critically ill patients is the Ramsay scale (Table 1).[21] Using a 6-point scale, from anxious and agitated (1) to completely unresponsive (6), this scale is widely considered to be the best of its type. It does have its drawbacks, however. As it is dependent on movement, modifications must be made when muscle relaxants are used. The sedation status of a patient may be unclear if they satisfy multiple criteria. An agitated patient who, at the same time, was only responsive to a light glabellar tap, could be rated as either a 1 or a 4.[11] There is also a lack of consensus as to what an appropriate target Ramsay score is. Some studies report levels of 2–4, while others use 4–6. Nevertheless, this scale has been used in 20 of 31 randomized controlled trials, has good inter-rater reliability, and an excellent correlation with the modified Glasgow Coma Scale (GCS).[15] Two other sedation scales, the Sedation-Agitation Scale (Table 2) and the Motor Activity Assessment Scale (MAAS) were mentioned in a recent review of sedation scoring systems and were felt to have similar degrees of inter-rater reliability and construct validity.[11]

Analgesia

As the national guidelines dictate,[24] the author recommends that pain in the ICU be treated with parenteral narcotics as first-line agents. Narcotics are central nervous system μ-receptor agonists that induce analgesia and, at higher doses, some degree of sedation, with other side effects listed below. The three agents to be used for ICU pain are morphine, fentanyl, and hydromorphone (in order of preference). As the pharmacodynamic (what the drug does to the body) profiles

TABLE 2. Sedation-Agitation Scale

Score	Description	Example
+3	Immediate threat to safety	Pulling at endotracheal tube or catheters, trying to climb over bedrail, striking at staff
+2	Dangerously agitated	Requiring physical restraints and frequent verbal reminding of limits, biting endotracheal tube, thrashing side-to-side
+1	Agitated	Physically agitated, attempting to sit up, calms down to verbal instructions
0	Calm and cooperative	Calm, arousable, follows commands
−1	Oversedated	Difficult to arouse or unable to attend to conversation or commands
−2	Very oversedated	Awakens to noxious stimuli only
−3	Unarousable	Does not awaken to any stimuli

of the aforementioned narcotics are similar, it is the pharmacokinetic (what the body does to the drug) properties that lead to the preference of one drug over another as an intravenous (IV) analgesic. The advantages and disadvantages of each of these agents and the appropriate dosing regimens are discussed.

Morphine

Parenteral narcotics should be used to control pain in the critically ill patient and morphine is considered the first-line agent. Clinicians have a great degree of familiarity with this drug, it is inexpensive, and has potency appropriate for the ICU. From a cardiac standpoint, morphine has the advantage of causing increases in both venous and arteriolar capacitance. Unfortunately, morphine also has negative characteristics, including histamine release, hypotension, and the potential to exacerbate respiratory depression and ileus. Morphine has a half-life of approximately 2 hours after IV injection, and a bolus of 0.05 mg/kg should be given, often followed by an IV infusion of 2–10 mg/hr.

Fentanyl

This drug, a synthetic opiate, is more potent and lipophilic than morphine. Therefore, it has a more rapid onset of action. In addition, fentanyl has the advantage of not releasing histamine and hence is an optimal drug to use if there

TABLE 3. Pharmacology of Intravenous Narcotics

Drug	Morphine	Fentanyl	Hydromorphone
Distribution half-life (min)	20	3	15
Elimination half life (hr)	2–4	2–5	2–4
Peak effect (min)	30	4	20
Equianalgesic dose (mg)	10	0.1	2
Suggested intravenous doses			
Bolus	2–5 mg	25–100 µg	0.5–1 mg
Infusion	2–10 mg/hr	25–100 µg/hr	0.5–2 mg/hr

are concerns about hemodynamic instability. Despite fentanyl's rapid onset and short half-life, it can accumulate in the peripheral compartment after prolonged infusion, increasing its half-life from 45 minutes to 9–16 hours. For those reasons, fentanyl should be reserved for ICU patients whose hemodynamic instability is a concern, in addition to situations involving a history of morphine allergy or histamine release with morphine. Loading doses are usually 1–2 µg/kg (25–100 µg) and continuous infusions are 1–2 µg/kg/hr (25–100 µg/hr).

Hydromorphone

Hydromorphone is an appropriate third-line agent for analgesia in the ICU. This semisynthetic opioid is 5–10-fold more potent than morphine. At therapeutic doses it appears to have minimal hemodynamic effect and does not result in the release of histamine. The bolus dose of hydromorphone is 0.5–1mg with infusion doses of 0.5–2 mg/hr.

Drugs to Avoid

Meperidine

For multiple reasons, meperidine is a poor choice for analgesia in the ICU setting. Firstly, a meperidine metabolite, normeperidine, lowers the seizure threshold. In addition, the drug has an atropine-like effect that can lead to tachycardia, has a fairly low potency, and can cause histamine release. Some authors, however, do recommend its use for shivering patients.[12]

NSAIDs

As a class, nonsteroidal anti-inflammatory drugs (NSAIDs) have no distinct advantage over narcotics with regards to ICU analgesia and have the potential for

TABLE 4. Pharmacology of Intravenous Benzodiazepines

Drug	Diazepam	Midazolam	Lorazepam
Distribution half-life (min)	10–15	7–10	3–10
Elimination half-life (hr)	20–40	2–2.5	10–20
Peak effect (min)	3–5	2–5	15–30
Equipotent dose (mg)	5	3	1
Suggested intravenous doses			
Bolus (mg)	5–10	0.5–2	0.5–2
Infusion (mg/kg/hr)	—	0.01–0.2	0.01–0.1

life-threatening side effects, such as gastrointestinal hemorrhage and renal failure. Therefore, this class of agent cannot be recommended for analgesia in the ICU.

Sedation in the ICU

Once the patient has received proper analgesia, and has had their sedation status evaluated, the next required step is parenteral sedative therapy. As set out in recent national guidelines from the Society of Critical Care Medicine,[24] the primary agents to be used are the benzodiazepines midazolam and lorazepam as well as the substituted isopropylphenol, propofol. For short-term sedation, midazolam and propofol have the most appropriate pharmacologic profile, while lorazepam is recommended for long-term sedation. These agents are considered in detail, indicating the appropriate dosages and clinical settings, as well as positive and negative attributes of each.

Pharmacokinetics of Continuous Infusions. In patients who are receiving prolonged IV infusions of sedatives, the elimination half-life is not the best predictor of the true time it takes for the drug to disappear from the body. In this situation, the rate with which the drug leaves the body is dependent on how long the agent has been infused. This relationship is described as the context-sensitive half-time and represents the time for the drug concentration to decrease by 50% after the end of a continuous infusion. Of note, lorazepam has a much greater context-sensitive half-time when compared with the other sedating agents, contributing to its use primarily as a long-term sedation agent.[26]

Midazolam

This drug is a water-soluble benzodiazepine that has a rapid onset of action (within 2 minutes) and a short half-life (1–4 hrs). The major side effect issues are those of hypoventilation and hypotension, especially in the setting of hypovolemia. Initial bolus doses vary by author, ranging from 0.5–2 mg to 1–5 mg or 0.03 mg/kg. IV infusions, often following multiple bolus doses, should be between 0.01 and 0.2 mg/kg/hr. However, as with all IV sedative infusions, the rate must be decreased and the degree of sedation of the patient must be checked, some authors recommend on a daily basis, as metabolites build up during the course of the infusion. Midazolam is considered to be the drug of choice for short-term sedation in the ICU, although it has a longer time to recovery when compared with propofol.

Lorazepam

Lorazepam is considered to be the drug of choice for long-term (> 24 hours) sedation in the ICU. Although its distribution half-life is similar to that of midazolam, its context-sensitive half-time is much greater than for the other sedating drugs, reflecting both its longer elimination half-life (10–20 hours) and higher receptor specificity. It is also less lipid-soluble than the other benzodiazepines, causing delayed movement across the blood–brain barrier and consequentially an increased time to peak effect when compared with other sedating agents. Bolus doses should be between 0.5 and 2 mg with infusion doses of 0.01–0.1 mg/kg/hr. Given the peak effect time of 15–30 minutes, however, some authors recommend starting with boluses of midazolam as the lorazepam infusion reaches a therapeutic level. It is fairly clear from the available data that lorazepam is appropriate only when long-term sedation is required. If rapid onset of sedation is necessary, another agent (preferably midazolam) must be used in concert, and lorazepam does not provide predictable arousal times, again leading to the choice of other agents for short-term sedation. Nevertheless, it is clearly a safe and cost-effective agent for long-term ICU sedation.[24]

Propofol

Propofol is a highly lipid-soluble IV anesthetic of the alkylphenol group. It is insoluble in water and is therefore supplied as a lipid emulsion. In can induce unconsciousness in 30 seconds with a dose of 2–2.5 mg/kg, but in low doses this drug can be used to cause sedation in the ICU patient. Recovery from a single injection occurs within 5–10 minutes. The pharmacokinetic profile of propofol is somewhat complex. Although long-term infusions result in significant intralipid accumulation and prolonged elimination half-life, in reality, clinical studies have demonstrated that after an 86-hour infusion, the mean time for a 50% reduction in serum levels was only 10 minutes.[1] The mechanism is most likely due to a rapid clearance from the plasma. For these reasons, it is recommended that propofol be administered only as an IV infusion when used as an ICU sedation agent at a dose of 0.5–3 mg/kg/hr.

Propofol is indicated when rapid sedation is needed, if the patient remains agitated despite other sedating agents, and if rapid and predictable arousal times are required. At this time, however, it is primarily to be used as a short-term sedative, primarily due to cost factors. Some precautions that must be remembered when using propofol are:

1. Because propofol can cause profound hypotension, many clinicians do not begin with a bolus dose, given the tendency towards hypotension, although most of the time this hypotension responds to fluid resuscitation.

2. Aseptic technique must be used at all times when handling this drug as there have been reports of infection associated with the lipid medium.[3]

3. Propofol is contraindicated in patients who have egg or soybean allergy.

4. Elevation of serum triglycerides has been noted in some patients receiving prolonged infusions of propofol.

5. Propofol should always been given via central access, as severe pain can be associated with its infusion through a peripheral catheter.

One of the major controversies with regards to propofol that has remained unresolved is whether it is truly associated with faster wake-up time and more rapid interval to extubation when compared with midazolam. The data from the literature are contradictory and although it appears that propofol is associated with shorter and more predictable arousal time,[8] this could only be demonstrated in deepley sedated patients in whom midazolam takes longer to wear off.[19]

Less Frequently Used Drugs

Diazepam

Although the oldest and least expensive of the benzodiazepines, its prolonged elimination half-life makes it an inappropriate agent for long-term ICU sedation and cannot be recommended to be used as such.

Ketamine

Recent national guidelines do not recommend the use of this agent as a sedative in the ICU.[24] This is based primarily on the fact that ketamine, a phencyclidine derivative, has many untoward side effects, including elevated blood pressure, heart rate and intracranial pressure (ICP) as well as increased airway secretions. In addition, emergence (vivid dreams and hallucinations) can be a problem up to 30% of the time. Nevertheless, given its rapid onset and short duration of action, doses of 0.5–1 mg/kg are recommended for short (5–20 min) ICU procedures (i.e., dressing changes in burn units). It may also be useful for asthmatics during mechanical ventilation as its sympathomimetic effects provide bronchodilatory support. Some authors advise pretreatment with atropine (to decrease airway secretions) and benzodiazepines (to help prevent emergence) prior to use of ketamine.

TABLE 5. Adverse Effects of Commonly Used Agents for ICU Sedation

	Drug Class	Adverse Effect
Directly related to drug	Opioids	Respiratory depression
		Nausea and vomiting
		Decreased gut motility
		Pruritus
		Urinary retention
		Hypotension
	Benzodiazepines	Respiratory depression
		Hypotension
		Erythema multiforme
	Phenothiazines/ butyrophenones	Extrapyramidal syndrome
		Cholestatic hepatitis
		Neuroleptic malignant syndrome
Related to sedated condition		Muscle atrophy
		Venous stasis/thrombosis
		Pressure damage to soft tissue
		Prolonged obtundation

Barbiturates

Although useful in the operating room for rapid induction of unconsciousness and used in the ICU to decrease ICP, the barbiturates (thiopental and pentobarbital) have several disadvantages that make them inappropriate for prolonged ICU sedation. Some of these include hypotension, myocardial depression, tachyphylaxis, poor amnestic effects, infectious complications, induction of microsomal enzymes, and decreased pain threshold.

Etomidate

Although this fast-acting, short-duration IV anesthetic is becoming the drug of choice for inducing unconsciousness in rapid-sequence intubation protocols (at a usual dose of 0.3 mg/kg), its long-term use has been associated with adrenocortical suppression[25] and cannot be recommended for prolonged use in the ICU.

Drugs for Delirium

Haloperidol

Delirium is a state of clouding of consciousness with reduced ability to appropriately respond to external stimuli. It is often manifest as a decreased level of consciousness, altered sensory perception, disorientation, incoherent speech, and disorganized thinking.[20] Often there is either a decrease or increase in psychomotor activity. Opiates and benzodiazepines, appropriate therapy for anxiety and agitation, can often paradoxically exacerbate delirium. The butyrophenone neuroleptic haloperidol is generally recommended as first-line therapy for delirium in the ICU. Although not approved by the FDA, the IV formulation of haloperidol is reported to be safe and effective and is the most appropriate delivery modality for the ICU setting. Standard dosing regimens recommend that haloperidol be given intravenously at a dose of 2–10 mg and to repeat this dose every 2–4 hours. The onset of effect begins between 30 and 60 minutes and lasts 4–8 hours. If, in order to control the delirium, the patient is requiring dosing more frequently than every 4 hours, a continuous infusion should be considered.[23] This should be started at 10 mg/hr and increased by 1 mg/hr every 20 minutes with repeat boluses of 5–10 mg being acceptable. Some of the adverse reactions associated with haloperidol use are QT prolongation which can lead to torsades de pointes (TDP), a reduction of the seizure threshold, and extrapyramidal (dystonic) reactions, the incidence of which can be reduced by using the IV form of the drug.

Controversies and Complications

Daily Awakening

Continuous infusions of intravenous sedation are commonplace in the modern ICU to promote patient comfort and facilitate the care of the patient by the nursing staff. Studies have shown, however, that prolonged continuous IV sedative infusions are independent risk factors for extended duration of mechanical ventilation,[14] the development of ventilator-associated pneumonia,[22] and protracted ICU and hospital stays. In addition, continuous intravenous sedation makes it difficult for clinicians to perform informative neurologic evaluations on ICU patients, potentially leading to costly and unnecessary neurologic imaging studies. A study of patients receiving continuous intravenous sedation was recently completed that compared outcomes of patients receiving standard care with those in whom the infusion was stopped on a daily basis.[16] On average, the patients who were awakened on a daily basis had two fewer days of mechanical ventilation and an ICU length of stay that was decreased by 3.5 days, as well as

TABLE 6. Cost Comparison of Common Sedative and Analgesic Agents

	Drug	$/Bottle	mg/Bottle	Daily Infusion Cost ($)
Analgesia	Morphine	12.50	500	6.00
	Fentanyl	0.40	0.1	9.60
Sedation	Propofol	15.28	500	308.04
	Midazolam	44.98	50	43.18
	Lorazepam	5.52	4	33.12

Wholesale costs for a large teaching institution.

a nearly 50% reduction in the dose of midazolam used. Despite these results, it is still unclear if this is to become the standard of care. The level of emotional and psychological distress of the patient (both at the time of the intervention and afterwards) was not measured, nor were the adverse cardiovascular effects of repeated sedative cessation. Another issue not addressed in this study was that of sedative withdrawal. A recent study examining this issue[7] showed that 32% of patients receiving sedation therapy for more than 1 week showed evidence of withdrawal (anxiety, vomiting or seizures) after gradual discontinuation of the infusion. Some are concerned that the result of this study may lead to more continuous ICU sedation as clinicians may develop a sense that by using daily awakening, they will prevent any unnecessary ICU time.[13] Further studies will need to be performed that take into account not only time of mechanical ventilation and length of stay in the ICU but psychological variables as well in order to best determine the medical validity of daily awakenings in the ICU.

Sedation Protocols

One of the problems that has emerged in the field of ICU sedation is that enormous variability exists among clinicians as to which drugs are chosen and how they are used to relieve pain and anxiety. As an attempt to solve this problem, recent studies have looked at the value of nursing-based protocols in the delivery of ICU analgesia and sedation. The theoretical advantages include the prevention of prescribing variability, enhancing the use of appropriate drugs, reducing drug costs, and even improving patient comfort. There are, however, very few studies rigorously analyzing the outcomes of sedation protocols, and the results are somewhat conflicting. One study shows a dramatic decrease in time of continuous intravenous sedation, duration of mechanical ventilation, time in ICU, and requirement for tracheostomy.[5] Another study only showed reduced drug costs and enhanced quality of sedation and analgesia.[18] However, the first study was much larger and better powered. It is not surprising, however, that at this time there is no clear answer as to the value of protocols in the delivery of ICU sedation, given that these studies used different protocols (each with slightly different pharmaceutical combinations and Ramsey scale targets). Although more studies will need to be performed to determine the optimal sedation protocol, it is clear even from this preliminary literature that sedation protocols appear to be safe and effective methods for improving the quality of analgesia and anxiolysis in the ICU.

Cost-Effective Sedation

Although the ICU usually accounts for approximately 10% of all inpatient beds, it can account for up to 25% of total hospital budgets. Of this, 25% of ICU costs are pharmacy costs and up to 15% can be related to purchasing sedatives, hypnotics, analgesics, and neuromuscular blocking agents.[10] Given the current economic environment in health care and concerns about rapidly escalating costs, the agent of choice for ICU sedation must not only have an appropriate pharmacologic profile and be proven safe, but it must be cost-effective as well.

Of the three principal sedating agents (propofol, midazolam, and lorazepam), propofol is clearly the most expensive in terms of drug acquisition costs. As these drugs have dramatically different pharmacokinetic/pharmacodynamic profiles, the determination of the overall cost of a particular agent cannot be based on the price of the drug alone and must include the cost of the compound itself plus drug delivery and nursing. Unfortunately, the results of recent studies attempting to look at overall sedation costs have not been in agreement with each other. This should not be surprising, however, given the variability in the indications for sedation and depth of sedation.

Nevertheless, a very recent randomized study looking at all three drugs found that sedation costs of propofol ($273/day) were greater than either midazolam ($182/day) or lorazepam ($48/day).[19] Although the authors felt that midazolam was the best agent overall in terms of percentage of patients who were appropriately sedated (rather than under- or oversedated), their final recommendations were for lorazepam given its cost-benefit ratio. Other studies, somewhat larger than the aforementioned, comparing propofol with midazolam demonstrated overall cost savings during sedation with propofol, primarily related to its rather short recovery time.[2] In addition, as the drugs go "off patent," their costs will drop by up to 50%. It is critical that ICU clinicians continue to work closely with their pharmaceutical counterparts so that they can incorporate cost-effectiveness data into their choice of ICU sedative.

Conclusions

Drug Choice

Each of the three drugs currently recommended for ICU sedation has a setting in which it is most appropriate, and no one drug is best for all situations given the profound variability in both patient pathophysiology and sedation requirements in the critical care environment.

Propofol is 3–4 times more expensive than the other two drugs and has the disadvantages of fairly frequent hypotension during bolus administration. It does, however, have the distinct advantages of rapid recovery time (as described above, some authors have shown that this may lead to an overall cost benefit) and should be used for short-term situations where a short, predictable wake-up time is required. Lorazepam has been recommended as the drug of choice by some authors given its cost-effectiveness profile. Others feel that as it has both a slow onset of action and a slow and often unpredictable recovery time, it should be used primarily when long-term sedation is required. This leaves midazolam, which more and more authors currently feel should be the first-line agent for short-term sedation in the ICU. Its only drawbacks are that it is less cost-effective for long-term sedation compared with lorazepam and it does not have as rapid a recovery time as propofol.

Intermittent Bolus vs. Continuous Administration

There are few data in the literature to support continuous intravenous sedation infusions as opposed to intermittent bolus as the preferred method for ICU sedation. However, from a practical standpoint, if a patient is receiving either narcotics or sedative injection more than every 2 hours, it is reasonable to begin a continuous intravenous infusion. As discussed above, however, infusions themselves appear to be associated with prolonged ICU stays and other adverse events. Recent studies have attempted to alleviate this problem with nurse-directed protocols and daily decreases of sedation to evaluate the mental and weaning status of the patient. The results from these studies appear to be positive, but there are concerns that they may come at the result of increased patient psychological discomfort.

Summary

Great strides have been made in the field of critical care medicine, allowing patients to survive illnesses they never would have even a few decades ago. Along with those advances, however, have come new challenges, such as combating the iatrogenic pain and suffering that can be all too common in the ICU setting. Using the guidelines above, the ICU clinician should be able to determine which agent or combination thereof can best assuage their patient's anxiety. As is often the case in clinical medicine, decisions with regard to sedation in the ICU must be made with a less than complete data set. The guiding principle of patient comfort, however, should be paramount at all times.

References

1. Bailie GR, Cockshott ID, Douglas EJ, et al: Pharmacokinetics of propofol during and after long-term continuous infusion for maintenance of sedation in ICU patients. Br J Anaesth 68:486–491, 1992.
2. Barrientos-Vega R, Mar Sanchez-Soria M, Morales-Garcia C, et al: Prolonged sedation of critically ill patients with midazolam or propofol: Impact on weaning and costs. Crit Care Med 25:33–40, 1997.
3. Bennett SN, McNeil MM, Bland LA, et al: Postoperative infections traced to contamination of an intravenous anesthetic, propofol. N Engl J Med 333:147–154, 1995.
4. Bergbom-Engberg I, Haljamae H: Assessment of patients' experience of discomfort during respirator therapy. Crit Care Med 17:1068–1072, 1989.
5. Brook AD, Ahrens TS, Schaiff R, et al: Effect of a nursing-implemented sedation protocol on the duration of mechanical ventilation. Crit Care Med 27:2609-15, 1999.
6. Cammarano W, Drasner K, Katz J: Pain control, sedation, and use of muscle relaxants. In Hall J, Schmidt G, Wood D (eds): Principles of Critical Care. New York, McGraw-Hill, 1997, pp 87–109.
7. Cammarano WB, Pittet JF, Weitz S, et al: Acute withdrawal syndrome related to the administration of analgesic and sedative medications in adult intensive care unit patients. Crit Care Med 26:676–684, 1998.
8. Carrasco G, Molina R, Costa J, et al: Propofol vs midazolam in short-, medium-, and long-term sedation of critically ill patients: A cost-benefit analysis. Chest 103:557–564, 1993.
9. Chapman CR, Casey KL, Dubner R, et al: Pain measurement: An overview. Pain 22:1–31, 1985.
10. Cheng EY: The cost of sedating and paralyzing the critically ill patient. Crit Care Clin 11:1005–1019, 1995.
11. De Jonghe B, Cook D, Appere-De-Vecchi C, et al: Using and understanding sedation scoring systems: A systematic review. Intensive Care Med 26:275–285, 2000.
12. Guffin A, Girard D, Kaplan JA: Shivering following cardiac surgery: Hemodynamic changes and reversal. J Cardiothorac Anesth 1:24–28, 1987.
13. Heffner JE: A wake-up call in the intensive care unit. N Engl J Med 342:1520–1522, 2000.
14. Kollef MH, Levy NT, Ahrens TS, et al: The use of continuous i.v. sedation is associated with prolongation of mechanical ventilation. Chest 114:541–548, 1998.
15. Kress JP, O'Connor MF, Pohlman AS, et al: Sedation of critically ill patients during mechanical ventilation: A comparison of propofol and midazolam. Am J Respir Crit Care Med 153:1012–1018, 1996.
16. Kress JP, Pohlman AS, O'Connor MF, et al: Daily interruption of sedative infusions in critically ill patients undergoing mechanical ventilation [see comments]. N Engl J Med 342:1471–1417, 2000.
17. Ledingham IM, Bion JF, Newman LH, et al: Mortality and morbidity amongst sedated intensive care patients. Resuscitation 16(Suppl):S69–S77, 1988.
18. MacLaren R, Plamondon JM, Ramsay KB, et al: A prospective evaluation of empiric versus protocol-based sedation and analgesia. Pharmacotherapy 20:662–672, 2000.

19. McCollam JS, O'Neil MG, Norcross ED, et al: Continuous infusions of lorazepam, midazolam, and propofol for sedation of the critically ill surgery trauma patient: A prospective, randomized comparison. Crit Care Med 27:2454–2458, 1999.
20. Nejman A: Sedation and Paralysis. In Civetta J, Taylor R, and Kirby R (eds): Critical Care, 3rd ed. Philadelphia, Lippincott-Raven, 1997, pp 821–836.
21. Ramsay MA, Savege TM, Simpson BR, et al: Controlled sedation with alphaxalone-alphadolone. Br Med J 2:656–659, 1974.
22. Rello J, Diaz E, Roque M, et al: Risk factors for developing pneumonia within 48 hours of intubation. Am J Respir Crit Care Med 159:1742–1746, 1999.
23. Riker RR, Fraser GL, Cox PM: Continuous infusion of haloperidol controls agitation in critically ill patients. Crit Care Med 22:433–440, 1994.
24. Shapiro BA, Warren J, Egol AB, et al: Practice parameters for intravenous analgesia and sedation for adult patients in the intensive care unit: An executive summary. Crit Care Med 23:1596–1600, 1995.
25. Wagner RL, White PF, Kan PB, et al: Inhibition of adrenal steroidogenesis by the anesthetic etomidate. N Engl J Med 310:1415–1421, 1984.
26. Young C, Knudsen N, Hilton A, et al: Sedation in the intensive care unit. Crit Care Med 28:854–866, 2000.

Procedural Sedation in the Emergency Department

6

Susan C. Lambe, M.D.

The optimal management of pain and anxiety is an important component of high-quality emergency care for patients of all ages. Pain control is often not adequately addressed in the emergency setting, for reasons including fear of oversedation, concern about altering physical findings, and underestimation of patient needs, especially at the extremes of age.[20] However, aggressive treatment of pain and anxiety improves quality of care and patient satisfaction by minimizing pain and facilitating procedures.

In the emergency department (ED) setting, the term procedural sedation is often used instead of conscious sedation. According to the American College of Emergency Physicians' Subcommittee on Procedural Sedation and Analgesia, procedural sedation describes "a technique ...intended to result in a depressed level of consciousness that allows the patient to tolerate unpleasant procedures [and is]... not likely to produce a loss of protective airway reflexes."[1] The term is thought to better reflect the spectrum of sedation, ranging from anxiety reduction to deeper states that might occur during procedures in the emergency department.

This chapter discusses indications for sedation, patient selection, recommended equipment and personnel, agents, and potential complications, as well as the appropriate post-procedure discharge for patients in the emergency department.

Indications for Emergency Procedural Sedation

Deciding whether a given clinical situation merits the use of procedural sedation can be difficult. Among other things, the physician must consider his or her familiarity with specific agents, experience with airway management, ED capabilities, hospital and ED protocols, and patient preparation. Adequate personnel with sufficient time to devote to the procedure are also essential.

TABLE 1. Clinical Indications for Sedation in the ED

Orthopedic reductions	Chest tube insertion
Cardioversion	Pediatric sexual assault exams
Wound debridement	Burn care
Pediatric laceration repair (e.g., tongue, eyelid, vermilion border)	CT scans and other diagnostic procedures in children
Lumbar puncture	Peritoneal lavage
Abscess incision and drainage	Removal of vaginal and rectal foreign bodies

In determining whether sedation is indicated, the physician must weigh the risks and benefits based on the clinical situation. For some procedures sedation is clearly justified, while other cases are more difficult, such as a pediatric laceration repair. For a simple extremity laceration, the risks might far outweigh any potential benefit. Conversely, for repair of a complex facial laceration, sedation might be essential. A partial list of indications for emergency procedural sedation is given in Table 1.

Patient Selection

Multiple factors must be taken into account in selecting patients for procedural sedation. Issues to consider include patient age, underlying medical problems, time since last meal, concurrent prescription and nonprescription

TABLE 2. Factors to Consider in Choosing an Agent for ED Sedation

Patient's age
Medical history
Time since last food or drink
Prior drug or alchol use
Agents given in the ED prior to procedure
Time constraints
Availability of equipment and personnel
Physician's familiarity with drugs
Indications and contraindications of specific agents

TABLE 3. American Society of Anesthesiologists Physical Status Classification

Category	Status
1	Healthy patient
2	Mild systemic disease (e.g., controlled COPD, hypertension, prior MI, diabetes)
3	Severe systemic disease (e.g., moderate COPD, coronary artery disease with angina)
4	Severe systemic disease that is a constant threat to life (e.g., marked CHF, unstable angina)
5	Moribund patient not expected to survive without the procedure

medications, physician time constraints, and availability of personnel and equipment (Table 2). Physician familiarity with various agents, their indications, and contraindications is also important. The clinician should be extremely cautious with unfamiliar agents, and ideally become familiar with them in a supervised environment prior to using them alone.

Emergent situations may require immediate intervention, but when patient stability permits, a thorough history and physical exam allows the physician to anticipate and prepare for potential complications. The history should include details of the indication for sedation, patient's volume status, associated injuries, drug or alcohol use, and medications given in the emergency department prior to sedation. Past medical history, allergies, current medications, and prior anesthesia information also should be obtained.

The risk of aspiration and time of last meal also must be considered. While no evidence-based guidelines exist for optimal fasting duration prior to sedation in the emergency department, it is logical to assume that risk of aspiration is lower with an empty stomach. In the absence of reliable ED data, the American Society of Anesthesiologists has recommended 6 hours NPO for solids and 2 hours for liquids.[2] The urgency of the procedure must be balanced against the risk associated with inadequate fasting. In the setting of life or limb threat, sedation should not be delayed to optimize NPO time, but practitioners must be prepared to deal with possible vomiting or aspiration. In elective situations, the practitioner should consider keeping the patient NPO for 2 hours (liquids) or 6 hours (solids) before sedation.

A targeted physical exam prior to sedation allows the physician to anticipate and prepare for potential complications. Assessment of vital signs, mental status, cardiorespiratory status and evaluation of the airway should occur before any elective procedure. ASA status should be determined. In general, ED sedation should be limited to ASA class 1 or 2 patients for non-emergent procedures (Table 3). For non-emergent cases with ASA class 3 or higher, consultation with an anesthesiologist is recommended. An important caveat is that ED sedation is for *brief* painful or unpleasant outpatient procedures. Any procedure requiring prolonged sedation is probably best performed by an anesthesiologist in the operating room.

Consent

In cases with no immediate threat to life or limb, it is good practice to discuss with patients all medications and interventions that will be provided. Discussion should include risks, benefits, potential side effects, and alternatives. Written or verbal consent should be obtained and this should be documented.

Procedural sedation and analgesia is sometimes necessary in situations when the patient is in severe pain or extremely anxious because of the circumstances surrounding the emergency visit. Such situations limit the patient's ability to fully consider issues discussed in the consent process. In other situations, the process is limited by an altered mental status, which impairs the patient's ability to understand risks and benefits. Sedation and analgesia under implied consent may be appropriate in these circumstances.[1]

Equipment and Personnel

The use of appropriate monitoring and personnel is essential to safe and effective delivery of sedation in the emergency department. While it would be optimal to have a designated sedation bed with monitors and drugs readily at hand, in nearly all facilities a resuscitation bed is used, and monitors and personnel are drawn from other areas of the department. The Joint Commission on Accreditation of Healthcare Organizations (JCAHO) mandates that standards for procedures within the hospital, such as sedation, must be uniform throughout the facility. The emergency department must maintain the same level of care, the same monitors and personnel, as the anesthesiologist provides in the operating room. While this may seem a daunting requirement, this standard ensures the same high quality of care for all patients.

Equipment for ED sedation falls into two categories: monitoring and resuscitative. Monitoring equipment includes noninvasive monitors such as electrocardiogram, blood pressure monitor, pulse oximeter, and capnograph, which allow continuous assessment of the patient during the procedure. Resuscitation equipment includes oxygen, suction, airway instruments, and reversal agents.

Monitoring Equipment

Because most untoward events that occur during outpatient sedation are related to inadequate monitoring,[13] it is absolutely critical the patient is thoroughly monitored. Adequate monitoring permits the physician to continuously monitor the status of the patient during the procedure. The degree of monitoring should be individualized depending on the situation. For example, a small dose of an opiate for analgesia does not warrant the same level of monitoring as a larger dose of a sedative-hypnotic agent.

Failure to recognize hypoxemia is clearly associated with an increase in complications.[17,21] The pulse oximeter allows early recognition of hypoxemia and has become the mainstay of monitoring for sedation in the emergency department. Pulse oximetry is recommended as the absolute minimum level of monitoring, appropriate for situations in which the patient is very unlikely to experience cardiorespiratory compromise.

Automated blood pressure monitoring also is very valuable. Setting the cycle for 1 minute allows close monitoring of the patient's hemodynamic status. Because fluctuations in blood pressure are most likely to occur while the agent is being titrated and during the first few minutes after the agent is given, monitoring should be most frequent during that period.

End-tidal carbon dioxide monitoring is another useful adjunct. A device that samples exhaled carbon dioxide provides a real-time respiratory waveform, reflecting the depth and rate of respiration during the procedure. This allows the physician to detect hypoventilation early in the course of the procedure, before hypoxia occurs.[11] Some systems have a port to connect to a nasal cannula to allow CO_2 sampling while oxygen is being delivered. Others require that an angiocath connected to a capnographer be placed through a nasal cannula prong. This allows close monitoring and permits early intervention in patients with compromised ventilatory status.

Continuous ECG monitoring provides real-time monitoring of the patient's heart rate. It allows the physician to detect any adverse cardiac effects and monitor the adequacy of sedation. An unexplained persistent tachycardia might reflect a response to pain, indicating inadequate analgesia. ECG monitoring also allows detection of infrequent arrhythmias that occur due to hypoxia, hypercarbia, or hypovolemia. The decision to use ECG monitoring depends on the agents employed, the individual patient, and standards for monitoring in other parts of the hospital.

Resuscitative Equipment

While adverse events are rare, procedural sedation may result in an allergic reaction, respiratory arrest or cardiac arrest. The likelihood of complications depends on the agent, dose and rate at which it is delivered, as well as individual patient characteristics. Equipment and trained personnel must be prepared to manage the airway, treat allergic reactions, drug overdoses, and cardiorespiratory compromise.

Suction, an oxygen source, an age-appropriate oral airway, and a bag-valve mask are essential for all procedures and should be readily available at the bedside. Ideally, patients should be pre-oxygenated for 5 minutes prior to the procedure. This creates a functional oxygen reservoir that reduces the risk of desaturation should a period of apnea occur. For simple procedures, a nasal cannula is sufficient. When using agents that induce a deeper level of sedation, such as methohexital, high-flow oxygen is advisable.

Airway equipment, including laryngoscopes, endotracheal tubes and stylettes must be at the bedside or easily accessible, depending on the clinical situation. Advanced life support equipment, including a defibrillator and a cardiac arrest cart with standard resuscitation drugs, should be available nearby in the emergency department. A reliable intravenous catheter is also highly advisable, depending on the agent, dose, and route of administration.[10]

Reversal agents, such as the opioid antagonist, naloxone, and the benzodiazepine antagonist, flumazenil, should be accessible whenever these drugs are used.[5] Ideally, the degree of sedation should be titrated to a level that optimizes patient analgesia and anxiolysis, but does not require reversal. Reversal can cause unpleasant side effects, such as emesis and pain. Also, reversal agents may have shorter half-lives than the sedating agents, requiring that patients be observed for a similar period even when reversal agents are used.

Personnel

Safe and effective delivery of procedural sedation requires emergency department personnel who have experience with the agents, the ability to monitor the patient's condition and recognize early signs of deterioration, and the skills to manage a compromised airway. If the individual performing the procedure is unable to continuously monitor the patient's airway, an additional provider dedicated to delivery of sedation should be present. Attempting to monitor a patient and simultaneously perform a procedure can be difficult and unsafe. The dedicated sedation provider should have no role in the performance of the procedure, and should only be responsible for administering the agents, observing the patient's airway, adequacy of ventilation, vital signs, and monitoring devices. This dedicated provider must be capable of recognizing and managing airway emergencies.

There are some situations where exceptions are acceptable, for example when low doses of pharmacologic agents are used and the physician is able to maintain continuous visual or verbal communication with the patient. However, even under these circumstances, the provider present must be capable of managing airway emergencies.

EMERGENCY DEPARTMENT
CONSCIOUS SEDATION DATA RECORD

MEDICAL RECORD NO.
PATIENT NAME
DATE OF BIRTH
WARD/UNIT   DATE

Date _____ wt (kg) _____ ht (in) _____ Allergies _____

T_____ BP_____ HR_____ RR_____

ASA class (Circle one)   1   2   E1   E2   E3   E4   E5

INDICATION: ☐ orthopedic reduction ☐ wound debridement ☐ burn care ☐ abscess I & D ☐ laceration repair
☐ chest tube ☐ 261 exam ☐ CT ☐ cardioversion ☐ other, specify: _____

PRESENT ILLNESS: Associated injuries?   ☐ no ☐ yes, specify: _____
Currently intoxicated with alcohol or drugs?   ☐ no ☐ yes, specify: _____
Sedation in ED prior to conscious sedation?   ☐ no ☐ yes, specify: _____
Pregnant?   ☐ no ☐ yes ☐ NA
Current URI?   ☐ no ☐ yes

NPO DURATION: Liquid: ☐ 0-2 hours*   ☐ 2-6 hours   ☐ > 6 hours
Solid: ☐ 0-2 hours*   ☐ 2-6 hours*   ☐ > 6 hours

ANESTHESIA HISTORY: Prior sedation/anesthesia?   ☐ no ☐ yes
Complications   ☐ no ☐ yes, specify: _____
Family history of anesthesia complications? ☐ unknown ☐ no ☐ yes, specify: _____

MEDICAL HISTORY: ☐ none ☐ asthma ☐ cardiac disease ☐ COPD ☐ glaucoma ☐ HTN
☐ kidney disease ☐ liver disease ☐ psych history ☐ seizure disorder ☐ other, specify: _____

HABITS: ☐ ETOH ☐ IVDU ☐ cocaine ☐ amphetamines ☐ tobacco

AGENT(S):   ☐ chloral hydrate ☐ diazepam ☐ etomidate ☐ fentanyl ☐ ketamine ☐ ketorolac ☐ lorazepam
☐ meperidine ☐ methohexital ☐ midazolam ☐ morphine ☐ thiopental ☐ other, specify: _____

PROCEDURE: Preoxygenated? ☐ yes ☐ no   Consent obtained? ☐ yes ☐ no, why? _____
Duration of conscious sedation** (min.)_____   Recovery time*** (min.)_____
Procedure start time_____am/pm   Procedure end time_____am/pm

COMPLICATIONS: ☐ none ☐ aspirations ☐ seizure ☐ apnea ☐ arrhythmia ☐ hypoxia ☐ hypotension
☐ laryngospasm ☐ other: _____

ASSESSMENT: Patient satisfaction?   ☐ good ☐ fair ☐ poor
Provider satisfaction?   ☐ good ☐ fair ☐ poor

COMMENTS:

Provider name (print)_____ Signature_____ Provider#_____
Provider level: _____R 4 _____R 3 _____R 2 _____R 1 _____PA/NP _____student

Attending name (print)_____ Signature_____ Provider#_____

*ASA class E patients only
**Time from beginning of sedation until at baseline mental status
***Period of monitored observation after procedure until at baseline mental status

MONITORS: ☐ ECG ☐ end tidal CO_2 ☐ BP ☐ Pulse-ox

EQUIPMENT AVAILABLE: ☐ O_2 ☐ suction ☐ defibrillator ☐ ET tube ☐ laryngoscope ☐ bag-valve-mask
☐ reversal agents _____

LEVEL OF CONSCIOUSNESS WHEN MONITORING DISCONTINUED:
Lifts head off gurney?   ☐ yes ☐ no   Stable vitals for 30 minutes post procedure? ☐ yes ☐ no
Baseline mental status? ☐ yes ☐ no   Recall of procedure?   ☐ yes ☐ no

RN Name (print)_____ Signature_____

MD to complete

RN to complete

Figure 1. Sample ED procedural sedation record. (Reproduced with permission of the Society for Academic Emergency Medicine.)

Documentation

For documentation purposes, a specific procedural sedation form promotes adequate preparation and quality assurance (Fig. 1).[15] In general, careful documentation of the patient's preprocedure status and clinical status during and after the procedure are recommended. The frequency with which vital signs are recorded should be individualized, depending on the clinical situation and the agents employed. When using agents that provide a deeper level of sedation, more frequent monitoring is advisable.

Agent Selection

To minimize complications and optimize patient satisfaction, it is critical to choose the appropriate agent and dose for the patient, administer the drug in the proper setting and evaluate the patient before, during, and after their use. The ideal agent provides amnesia, analgesia, and anxiolysis. It is titrable, reversible, with rapid onset and offset, has a large therapeutic index, minimal effect on hemodynamics, and preserves protective airway reflexes. While no single agent provides all these properties, the provider must consider the relative strengths and weaknesses of a given agent with the clinical scenario, available equipment and personnel, and familiarity with the agent.

Each patient responds differently to drug administration. For example, an injection drug user may require a much higher dose of opiates than an elderly patient for the same procedure. Titration of the agent to patient response is extremely important. Physician familiarity with each pharmacologic profile also is critical. The following section is a summary of commonly used agents.

Opiates

Morphine, meperidine, and fentanyl are the most common opiates used in the ED. For some procedures, an opiate alone provides adequate analgesia and sedation. For others, an opiate is used in combination with an anxiolytic agent, such as midazolam or methohexital. Opiates are frequently used for procedural sedation, because they have a proven track record, predictable performance, reversibility, and are relatively inexpensive.

Of the opiates, fentanyl is extremely well-suited for use in the emergency department. It has a rapid onset and offset, high potency, rapid reversal with opiate antagonists, and minimal effect on hemodynamics. This unique combination of potency and short half-life permits administration of multiple small doses that can be easily titrated to desired clinical effect. Unlike other narcotics, fentanyl induces little histamine release and is seldom associated with hypotension. Anesthetic doses of fentanyl vary, but range from 50–100 mg/kg. In contrast, appropriate doses of fentanyl for emergency sedation are much lower, ranging from 1–5 mg/kg.

Adverse effects due to fentanyl are rare in the emergency department. They include hypotension, respiratory depression, muscular and glottic rigidity, seizures, generalized pruritus, and nausea and vomiting. In one series, respiratory depression and hypotension were more likely to occur in association with alcohol intoxication.[4] Mild side effects, including facial pruritus and nausea were more common. A rigid chest wall phenomenon is extremely rare and is associated with rapid infusion of higher doses, typically in excess of 15 mg/kg. This dose is significantly higher than is commonly used for procedural sedation.

Benzodiazepines

Benzodiazepines are frequently used for sedation in the emergency department. Their sedative and amnestic properties make them an excellent choice for anxiety-provoking procedures. When used alone, they provide no analgesia; however, when used with an opiate analgesic, they are effective for brief, painful procedures, such as fracture reduction or abscess incision and drainage.

Of the benzodiazepines, midazolam is used most often for emergency sedation because of its shorter onset and duration of action. When administered intravenously, it has an onset of approximately 1–3 minutes and a duration of action of 60 minutes.[16] It provides amnesia and sedation, but has no analgesic properties. Midazolam is water-soluble, which allows for oral, rectal, and intranasal use. These alternative routes are sometimes used for procedures in children, and produce a longer onset and duration of action than intravenous administration.

Early reports of complications from midazolam in the outpatient setting are thought to have been due to inadequate monitoring. As with all benzodiazepines, respiratory depression and hypotension are the most common complications. However, in a well-monitored emergency department setting, the complication rate is less than 1%.[22] Geriatric patients may be more susceptible to these effects; therefore, dosing should be adjusted accordingly.[16] Both hypotension and respiratory depression are reversed with flumazenil.[3]

Barbiturates

Barbiturates are sedative-hypnotic agents often used for induction of general anesthesia. Their rapid onset and short duration of action make them effective agents for short procedures in the emergency department. They provide brief sedation, but no analgesia. When used in combination with an analgesic, they are an excellent choice for short, painful procedures.

Methohexital is the barbiturate most often used for procedural sedation in the emergency department. The onset of action is 5–15 seconds and the duration of effect is 5–10 minutes. Methohexital provides excellent sedation and amnesia for very brief procedures, such as cardioversion or orthopedic reduction.

Adverse effects include respiratory depression and even apnea in a small percentage of patients.[23] Methohexital may cause hypotension and should be used with caution in patients with suspected hypovolemia. Some authors recommend that methohexital be avoided in patients with seizure disorders or a history of bronchospasm.[23]

Ketamine

Structurally related to phencyclidine, ketamine is a short-acting, dissociative anesthetic agent that produces amnesia, analgesia, and sedation. During sedation, patients become trance-like and unresponsive to stimuli, including pain. Skeletal muscle hypertonicity is seen, with random movements of the head or extremities, unrelated to painful stimuli. Airway reflexes, such as cough and gag, are preserved and may be exaggerated. Spontaneous respiration is not depressed and cardiorespiratory reflexes are maintained. Ketamine inhibits uptake of catecholamines, causing pupilary dilation, mild bronchodilation, and a transient rise in pulse and blood pressure.

Onset and duration of action varies with the route of administration. When given intramuscularly, onset is within 2–5 minutes and duration is 20–30 minutes. With intravenous administration, onset is approximately within 30 seconds and duration of action is 5–15 minutes. Clinical efficacy is apparent when nystagmus is observed.

Ketamine has a well-documented safety record for emergency department sedation for intravenous[5,9] and intramuscular[7,10] routes. It is an extremely safe and effective agent for short and intermediate-length procedures, such as pediatric fracture reduction and laceration repair. The most common adverse effect is the emergence phenomenon, a state characterized by bizarre hallucinations, nightmares, and dysphoria on awakening. This occurs in 0–50% of adults and 0–15% of children, and for this reason is more often used in pediatric patients. The emergence phenomenon can be blunted by maintaining a calm, quiet environment during the procedure and administration of a benzodiazepine on awakening. Ketamine causes an increase in oropharyngeal secretions, which is especially common in children. Some practitioners pretreat patients with atropine or glycopyrrolate to reduce the degree of hypersalivation. However, ketamine has been used extensively without these adjuncts with no consistently demonstrated increase in adverse events. Approximately 10% of patients will vomit after recovery. The emesis is generally brief, but the clinician should be aware of this when counseling parents. Laryngospasm and respiratory depression are uncommon side effects, which are typically self-limited and managed with bag-valve mask ventilation. Ketamine should be avoided in neonates, patients with increased intraocular or intracranial pressure, psychosis, coronary artery disease, pregnancy, hyperthyroidism, or hypertension.

Etomidate

Etomidate is a nonbarbiturate, ultrashort-acting imidazole derivative, structurally unrelated to other sedative hypnotic agents.[8] It causes sedation and hypnosis via the GABA receptors within the central nervous system. While it has not been studied extensively in the emergency department, etomidate has great potential for use in procedural sedation because of its rapid onset and short duration of action. Because it does not cause histamine release, etomidate has no clinically significant effect on cardiovascular tone. It is an excellent agent for patients with limited cardiac reserve. Compared with thiopental, etomidate causes less respiratory depression and has a shorter recovery time. Like other sedative-hypnotics, it provides no analgesia when used alone.

The recommended dose for procedural sedation is 0.1 mg/kg administered intravenously over 1 minute.[6] Onset of action occurs within about 1 minute, and sedation lasts approximately 5–10 minutes.

Etomidate may cause pain on injection, myoclonic jerks, and dose-dependent inhibition of corticosteroid synthesis. Although cortisol suppression is well-documented, one-time administration does not appear to lead to inadequate stress responses and does not appear likely to be a clinically significant concern for most emergency department patients.[6] Etomidate is not currently approved for use during pregnancy and for children under 12 years of age.

Propofol

An ultrashort-acting sedative-hypnotic, propofol provides sedation and amnesia, but no analgesia. Propofol is typically given as a bolus followed by a continuous infusion. It is an excellent choice for brief, invasive procedures in otherwise healthy patients. Propofol has inherent antiemetic effects and has been used in chemotherapy and ocular surgery.

Adverse effects include transient apnea, burning at the injection site, and hypotension. Because of the cardiovascular effects, it is recommended that propofol be used with caution in patients with compromised cardiovascular

TABLE 4. Criteria for Discontinuation of Monitoring

Return to baseline mental status
Stable hemodynamics and oxygenation for 30 minutes post-procedure
Ability to lift head off gurney
Respiratory status not compromised
No new signs, symptoms, or problems

Sample Discharge Instructions after Sedation/Analgesia

The medicines you have received in the emergency department can sometimes cause confusion, sleepiness, or clumsiness; therefore, you need to be extra careful for the next 24 hours. If you have any questions, please do not hesitate to call the emergency department.

For Children:
1. Do not leave the child unattended at any time in a car seat; if the child falls asleep in the car seat, watch the child continuously to make sure that he or she does not have any difficulty breathing.
2. No eating or drinking for at least the next 2 hours, and the child is completely awake and alert, and has no nausea. If the child is an infant, half a normal feeding may be given 1 hour after discharge.
3. If sleepy, the child should not be left alone, and should be awakened from sleep every hour for the next 4 hours. If the child's breathing does not appear normal to you or if you are unable to wake the child up, call 911, or return to the hospital *immediately.*
4. No playing that requires coordination (bikes, skating, swing sets, climbing, monkey bars, etc.) for the next 24 hours since these activities might result in the child injuring himself or herself.
5. No swimming or using machines that might cause injury for the next 24 hours without adult supervision.
6. Supervise all playing or bathing for the next 8 hours.
7. Return immediately to the emergency department for vomiting more than once, strange or unusual behavior, or any other symptom that does not seem normal for the child.

For Adults:
1. Do not engage in any activity that requires alertness or coordination for the next 24 hours. This includes: No driving, operating heavy machinery, using power tools, cooking, climbing, or riding a bicycle.
2. No swimming, hot tubs, or baths for the next 24 hours.
3. Remain in the company of a family member, friend, or attendant for the next 24 hours.
4. Do not make any important decisions in the next 24 hours, such as signing contracts, expensive purchases, important commitments, and so on.
5. No alcohol for 24 hours.
6. Do not eat or drink if you have any nausea.
7. Take only medications prescribed by your physician, in the dose prescribed.
8. Return to the emergency department for vomiting more than once, strange or unusual behavior, confusion, or any other worrisome symptoms.

Figure 2. Sample discharge instructions. (Reproduced with permission of the American College of Emergency Physicians.)

function, especially in the elderly and hypovolemic patients. When apnea occurs, it is very brief (usually < 30 seconds) and dose-dependent.[19] Pain on injection is minimized by using an antecubital vein and concomitant administration of lidocaine. In a double-blind comparison with midazolam in pediatric emergency patients, propofol provided equivalently effective sedation, more rapid recovery, and a similarly low rate of complications.[12] Propofol should be avoided in

TABLE 5. Discharge Criteria

Normal vital signs
Baseline mental status
Able to sit unassisted
Minimal nausea/able to take fluids by mouth
Pain and discomfort have been addressed

patients with allergies to egg, lecithin, or soybean oil, as these are constituents of the product's emulsion base.

Recovery and Disposition

Close monitoring during recovery is as crucial as it is during sedation. After the painful stimulus of the procedure is removed, patients are vulnerable to becoming more sedated with potential for airway and hemodynamic compromise. Personnel should remain with the patients and observe them until they are fully recovered. While each facility should develop individual policies for discharge after sedation, criteria for discontinuation of monitoring should include the ability to lift the head off the gurney, return to baseline mental status, and stable hemodynamics and oxygenation for 30 minutes after the procedure (Tables 4 and 5). If reversal agents are used, the observation period should be longer, as resedation can occur.[14,18]

References

1. American College of Emergency Physicians: Clinical policy for procedural sedation and analgesia in the emergency department. Ann Emerg Med 31:663–677, 1998.
2. American Society of Anesthesiologists: Practice guidelines for sedation and analgesia by non-anesthesiologists. Anesthesiology 84:459–471, 1996.
3. Chudnofsky CR: Safety and efficacy of flumazenil in reversing conscious sedation in the emergency department. Acad Emerg Med 4:944–949, 1997.
4. Chudnofsky CR, Wright SW, Dronen SC, et al: The safety of fentanyl use in the emergency department. Ann Emergn Med 18:635–639, 1989.
5. Dachs RJ, Innes GM: Intravenous ketamine sedation of pediatric patients in the emergency department. Ann Emerg Med 29:146–150, 1997.
6. Dursteler BB, Wightman JM: Etomidate-facilitated hip reduction in the emergency department. Am J Emerg Med 18:204–208, 2000.
7. Epstein FB: Ketamine dissociative sedation in pediatric emergency medical practice. Am J Emerg Med 11:180–182, 1993.
8. Giese JL, Stanley TH: Etomidate: A new intravenous anesthetic induction agent. Pharmacotherapy 3:251–258, 1983.
9. Green SM, Rothrock SG, Harris T, et al: Intravenous ketamine for pediatric sedation in the emergency department: Safety profile with 156 cases. Acad Emerg Med 5:971–976, 1998.
10. Green SM, Rothrock SG, Lynch EL, et al: Intramuscular ketamine for pediatric sedation in the emergency department: Safety profile in 1,022 cases. Ann Emerg Med 31:688–697, 1998.
11. Hart LS, Berns SD, Houck CS, et al: The value of end-tidal CO_2 monitoring when comparing three methods of conscious sedation for children undergoing painful procedures in the emergency department. Pediatr Emerg Care 13:198–193, 1997.
12. Havel CJ, Strai RT, Hennes H: A clinical trial of propofol vs. midazolam for procedural sedation in a pediatric emergency department. Acad Emerg Med 6:989–997, 1999.

13. Holzman, RS, Cullen DJ, Eichhorn JH, et al: Guidelines for sedation by non-anesthesiologists during diagnostic and therapeutic procedures. J Clin Anesth 6:265–276, 1994.

14. Innes G, Murphy M, Nijssen-Jordan C, et al: Procedural sedation and analgesia in the emergency department: Canadian consensus guidelines. J Emerg Med 17:145–156, 1999.

15. Koenig KL, Lambe SC: A model emergency department systemic sedation record. Acad Emerg Med 4:1178–1180, 1997.

16. Nordt SP, Clar RF: Midazolam: A review of therapeutic uses and toxicity. J Emerg Med 15:357–365, 1996.

17. Santos LJ, Varon J, Pic-Aluas L, et al: Practical uses of end-tidal carbon dioxide monitoring in the emergency department. J Emerg Med 12:633–644, 1993.

18. Shannon M, Albers G, Burkhart K, et al: Safety and efficacy of flumazenil in the reversal of benzodiazepine-induced conscious sedation. J Pediatr 131:582–586, 1997.

19. Swanson ER, Seaberg DC, Mathias S: The use of propofol for sedation in the emergency department. Acad Emerg Med 3:234–238, 1996.

20. Wilson J, Pendleton J: Oligoanalgesia in the emergency department. Am J Emerg Med 7:620–623, 1989.

21. Wright SW: Conscious sedation in the emergency department: The value of capnography and pulse oximetry. Ann Emerg Med 21:551–555, 1992.

22. Wright SW, Chudnofsky CR, Dronen SC, et al: Midazolam use in the emergency department. Am J Emerg Med 8:97–100, 1990.

23. Zink BJ, Darfler K, Salluzzo RF, et al: The efficacy and safety of methohexital in the emergency department. Ann Emerg Med 20:1293–1298, 1991.

7

Sedation of Pediatric Patients

Andrew Infosino, M.D.

Every day countless children are sedated by nonanesthesiologists for procedures outside the operating room because these procedures are either painful or frightening. Children often require sedation for procedures that are performed on adults without sedation because they are unable to remain immobile for extended periods of time and are often unwilling to cooperate with painful or uncomfortable procedures. Ideally, the sedation of children, even for procedures outside the operating room, would be performed by pediatric anesthesiologists, as they possess knowledge of the pharmacology of sedative and anesthetic medications as well as expertise in airway management and resuscitation skills. Realistically, the majority of children are sedated by nonanesthesiologists for procedures outside the operating room, for both economic and logistical reasons. Therefore, the goal of this chapter is to provide a framework for the nonanesthesiologist to safely provide sedation for children and to delineate which children should be referred to pediatric anesthesiologists for sedation and anesthesia.

There has been an increase in both the number and complexity of procedures being performed on children outside the operating room setting and many predict that in the future an increasing percentage of these procedures will be performed outside the traditional hospital setting. The hospital locations where children are routinely sedated include the emergency room for procedures such as suturing lacerations or setting fractures, the cardiac catheterization laboratory, the gastroenterology suite for endoscopies, interventional radiology, nuclear medicine, and various radiologic imaging areas, including ultrasound, magnetic resonance imaging (MRI), and computed tomography (CT). Locations outside the hospital where children are routinely sedated include free-standing surgery centers, dental offices, and free-standing radiologic imaging centers.

The sedation of children is difficult because they are often uncooperative with painful or frightening procedures and they often require a deeper level of sedation than an adult for the same procedure. The levels of sedation are in a

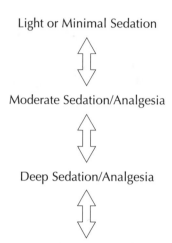

Figure 1. The continuum of sedation.

continuum with each other and with general anesthesia (Fig. 1). Many medical societies and organizations have attempted to accurately define the levels of sedation and to correlate appropriate levels of monitoring, competency, and certification of personnel to the level of sedation. Because there is a continuum of sedation with anesthesia it is impossible to guarantee that a "conscious," light," or "minimal" sedation does not become a "deep" sedation or general anesthesia (Table 1). The particular drug chosen to sedate a child or the route of administration also do not guarantee that only a particular level of sedation will be achieved, as there is tremendous variability in effect from patient to patient. In children it is extremely difficult to provide adequate sedation without the potential for the loss of protective airway reflexes or the occurrence of hypoventilation, apnea, airway obstruction, and the potential for respiratory or cardiac arrest. From the viewpoint of patient safety, it is imperative to treat all sedation in pediatric patients as deep sedation or anesthesia. This philosophy of maximizing patient safety requires the use of personnel who are competent and appropriately trained to sedate pediatric patients. To maximize patient safety it is also vital to adhere to proper presedation patient evaluations and NPO guidelines, to use appropriate monitoring during the sedation and to have all necessary pediatric equipment readily available.

It is important to recognize that the goals for sedating a pediatric patient may be different than for sedating an adult patient. In general, most adults can remain immobile for reasonable periods of time for such studies as MRIs, CT, nuclear medicine studies or even more invasive studies, such as cardiac catheterization. Pediatric patients are usually much less cooperative and will require sedative

TABLE 1. Definition of Levels of Sedation

Light or Minimal Sedation (Anxiolysis): A drug-induced state of depressed consciousness in which patients can respond normally to verbal commands. Patients can maintain and protect their airway and their ventilatory and cardiovascular functions are unaffected.

Moderate Sedation/Analgesia: A drug-induced state of depressed consciousness during which patients respond purposefully to verbal commands, either alone or accompanied by light tactile stimulation. Patients usually maintain and protect their airway. Ventilatory and cardiovascular functions may be slightly decreased, but remain adequate.

Deep Sedation/Analgesia: A drug-induced state of depressed consciousness from which patients cannot be easily aroused, but still respond purposefully to painful stimulation. Patients may not maintain an adequate airway and may not be able to protect their airway. Ventilatory function may be inadequate and the patients may require ventilatory assistance. Cardiovascular function may be slightly decreased, but remains adequate.

General Anesthesia: A drug-induced state of depressed consciousness from which patients are not arousable, even by painful stimulation. Patients often lose their ability to maintain and protect their airway. Ventilatory function is often inadequate and positive-pressure ventilation may be required because of depressed spontaneous ventilation or drug-induced depression of neuromuscular function. Cardiovascular function may be inadequate.

agents to ensure immobility. Analgesia can often be provided with local anesthesia, but children often require sedation before the injection of local anesthesia can be given. Whereas adults often only require a slight degree of anxiolysis for a procedure, children more commonly require complete sedation. Finally, amnesia is also a goal of pediatric sedation, to ensure that remembering the experience as painful or unpleasant will not emotionally traumatize the child. These differences in pediatric and adult sedation goals underscore why it is so difficult to provide "minimal," "light," or "conscious" sedation in pediatric patients.

Patient Evaluation

Every pediatric patient undergoing sedation should be evaluated with an appropriate history and physical examination in order to reduce the risk of adverse outcomes. This history and physical exam should be documented in the patient's medical record prior to sedating the patient. The pre-sedation evaluation is important because it may identify potential problems and may affect the choice of medications for sedation as well as identify which patients should be referred to a pediatric anesthesiologist for sedation.

The history should include a review of the major organ systems focusing primarily on the cardiac and pulmonary systems. Patients with a history of gastroesophageal reflux should be identified and if necessary should have their airways protected by endo-tracheal intubation for the procedure. An important question that is often overlooked is whether or not the child snores, as snoring can indicate the presence of obstructive sleep apnea. Children with obstructive sleep apnea are at particular risk for airway obstruction during sedation and in the majority of cases should be referred to a pediatric anesthesiologist. Children with a history of weakness or hypotonia being referred for sedation for a procedure such as a MRI are also at very high risk for airway obstruction and inadequate ventilation during sedation and should be sedated very cautiously or referred to a pediatric anesthesiologist. A history of any allergies to medications as well as a list of the medications the patient is taking should be included in the pre-sedation evaluation. As latex allergy is becoming increasingly prevalent, it is important to remember to question all pediatric patients regarding any possible latex allergy. Any patient with a history of any type or reaction to latex should be sedated with scrupulous avoidance of any latex-containing product. In patients with a history of severe or anaphylactic reactions to latex, it would be prudent to pretreat patients with diphenhydramine and steroids and to have epinephrine readily available in an appropriate dose for the patient. Any history of problems with a previous sedation or anesthetic should alert the practitioner to potential problems with the current sedation. The history should also include documentation of the last intake of solids and of clear liquids (see NPO guidelines below).

The physical exam, like the history, should be focused on the cardiac and pulmonary systems as well as an evaluation of the airway. Vital signs, including blood pressure, heart rate, and respiratory rate should be documented on the pre-sedation evaluation chart as well as a current weight and an oxygen saturation, measured while the child is breathing room air (unless the child requires supplemental oxygen). The airway exam begins with an evaluation of the body habitus, as obesity can often indicate potential airway problems, especially if the obesity involves the face and/or neck. The mouth should be evaluated for mouth opening and the presence of any loose teeth or an abnormally large tongue (macroglossia). A small mandible (micrognathia) can indicate potential difficulties with airway obstruction during sedation and difficulties with endotracheal intubation. The neck should be evaluated for flexion and extension. The heart should be auscultated to ensure that no murmurs are present and the lungs should be evaluated for any possible wheezing, rhonchi, rales, or respiratory distress. The majority of pediatric patients presenting for sedation require no laboratory studies.

TABLE 2. Fasting Guidelines for Infants and Children Prior to Sedation and/or Anesthesia

Clear liquids	2 hours
Breast milk	4 hours
Formula, non-clear liquids, and solids	6 hours

The pre-sedation evaluation should alert the practitioner to potential problems and should identify patients who should be referred to a pediatric anesthesiologist for sedation or anesthesia. Obviously, children who have had problems with a previous sedation or who have failed a previous sedation fall into this category. Children who are obese, weak, hypotonic, or who have airway anomalies or obstructive sleep apnea should also be referred to pediatric anesthesiologists.

The pre-sedation evaluation should also include documentation of a discussion of the risks and benefits of the sedation with the parents or guardian as well as consent from the parents or guardians to proceed with the sedation and the procedure.

NPO Guidelines

Regardless of the procedure or choice of sedative drugs, all children undergoing sedation should follow appropriate fasting guidelines prior to their procedure. As light sedation is on a continuum with deep sedation and anesthesia, the same NPO guidelines should be applied to pediatric patients for all levels of sedation as for anesthesia. There has been a gradual liberalization of NPO guidelines for children in order to make them more comfortable and at least allow them to drink clear liquids at a closer interval prior to the procedure. The American Society of Anesthesiologists has just published its current practice guidelines for preoperative fasting and these guidelines should be followed (Table 2).

The major reason why NPO guidelines need to be stringently adhered to is that even with light sedation, protective airway reflexes can be lost and the patient can aspirate stomach contents. In certain patients who have a higher risk of aspiration, more conservative NPO guidelines can be adopted. In children who emergently need sedation and did not fast appropriately, everything possible should be done to minimize the risk of aspiration. Neutralizing gastric acid with antacids should be considered, but a better approach may be to protect the airway from aspiration by placing an endotracheal tube after a rapid sequence induction with cricoid pressure by appropriately trained personnel.

Equipment, Monitoring, and Documentation

A successful sedation involves both proper equipment and monitoring. Prior to beginning any sedation, it is important to check that equipment is both available and functioning. Suction should be immediately available to deal with airway secretions as well as possible emesis. A method of delivering supplemental oxygen and positive-pressure ventilation is mandatory and a second, "back-up" oxygen source should always be immediately available. Supplemental oxygen should always be used during pediatric sedation. If the patient is cooperative enough, supplemental oxygen via nasal canula or face mask should be initiated prior to beginning the sedation. In children who will not tolerate supplemental oxygen while awake and alert, supplemental oxygen should be immediately available and should be initiated as soon as the child is sedated enough to tolerate it.

Resuscitation equipment, including a pediatric crash cart with an assortment of appropriately sized pediatric masks, endotracheal tubes, laryngeal mask airways, nasal and oral airways, laryngoscopes, and blades needs to be readily available. Equipment for starting an intravenous (IV) administration, including pediatric-sized IV catheters is also necessary. Drugs for sedating the patient and appropriate resuscitation drugs, including epinephrine, calcium, atropine, bicarbonate, lidocaine, and glucose should be available. If narcotics are being used to sedate the patient, the narcotic antagonist naloxone should be immediately available. Likewise, if benzodiazepines are being used to sedate the patient, the benzodiazepine antagonist flumazenil should be readily available.

Appropriate monitors are essential to patient safety during sedation. Many locations in which children are sedated today preclude the practitioner from directly being in contact with the patient. For example, a child in the MRI scanner is physically remote from the practitioner, necessitating appropriate remote monitoring. Other locations, such as endoscopy suites or cardiac catheterization laboratories, often have the lights dimmed to enable better visualization during the study, which makes it more difficult to directly observe the patient. At a minimum, blood pressure monitoring and pulse oximetry should be used. The pulse oximiter provides information about the adequacy of oxygenation and the heart rate and gives some basic information about whether the heart rhythm is regular or irregular. In pediatric patients without a history of heart disease, EKG, while important, is not as essential a monitor as pulse oximetry. If temperature monitoring is available, it should be used and every effort should be made to prevent hypothermia, especially in infants and small children. The room temperature should be increased and the infant or child should be covered with blankets or drapes, if possible.

As most sedative and anesthetic drugs depress ventilation, ventilation should be monitored continuously during the sedation. The best monitor is capnography or end-tidal carbon dioxide monitoring and should be used if available. The end-tidal CO_2 monitor can be connected to an endotracheal tube, laryngeal mask airway (LMA), or even a nasal canula or placed within a face mask. Capnography provides breath-by-breath information on the respiratory rate and provides instant notification if the airway is lost or compromised. It also provides indirect evidence of the depth of sedation and the depth of ventilatory compromise by providing an end-tidal CO_2 value. Significant elevations of end-tidal CO_2 above the normal baseline of 40 mmHg can indicate excessive sedation and the need for ventilatory support before respiratory arrest occurs.

If continuous end-tidal CO_2 monitoring is not available, breath sounds should be auscultated continuously with a precordial stethoscope or respiratory activity should be directly observed. If the situation precludes direct observation of the patient, video cameras often can be used to aid in remotely monitoring the patient from a distance.

If at all possible, an initial set of vital signs, oxygen saturation, and end-tidal CO_2 should be obtained and recorded on the sedation chart. If the child is uncooperative it may be necessary to begin the sedation and then initiate appropriate monitoring. A sedation record should be maintained throughout the procedure, recording the patient's vital signs, oxygen saturation, and end-tidal CO_2 value and should be continued until the patient has returned to his or her pre-sedation baseline. This recovery period should be either in the same location as the procedure or in a designated recovery area with appropriately trained personnel and equipment. The recovery area should be equipped similarly to the sedation area, with suction, oxygen sources, and a pediatric crash cart with appropriate pediatric-sized resuscitation equipment.

Personnel

The key to successful and safe sedation of pediatric patients is to ensure that the personnel responsible for sedating children is both competent and comfortable working with children. To ensure patient safety, there must be one person whose sole responsibility is to both sedate and monitor the patient during the procedure. This person should not be the person who is actually performing the procedure. The person providing sedation must be competent in sedation techniques and capable of managing potential complications associated with these techniques. At a minimum this person needs to be trained and certified in pediatric basic life support and ideally also trained and certified in pediatric advanced life support (PALS). During the procedure, the person sedating the pediatric patient would record and document the dosage, route, and time of all drugs given and the type and amount of IV fluids, and would record vital signs, oxygen saturation, and, if possible, end-tidal CO_2 on a regular basis on the sedation record.

The Practice of Sedating Pediatric Patients

The ideal method of sedating pediatric patients would be a medication given by mouth, or even better, absorbed through the skin, which would reliably sedate the patient without any respiratory depression or other side effects. This ideal medication would last exactly the length of the procedure or could be immediately reversed at the end of the procedure returning the patient to the pre-sedation status. Unfortunately, no such medication exists and all current sedation drugs have significant limitations and side effects.

Sedative medications can be given orally, intranasally, rectally, via subcutaneous or intramuscular injection, transdermally, intravenously, or can be absorbed via the lungs. While oral medications appear to be the simplest to administer to infants and children, there are several limitations of oral medications for sedation. Orally administered medications can exhibit a wide variability in absorption from patient to patient. The combination of the fact that most sedative medications are not available in a liquid form that tastes good and the fact that children are notorious for being poor medicine takers and often spit out medications, makes it very difficult to reliably administer an exact oral dose to a child. Additionally, once a child is given an oral dose of sedative medication, and for whatever reason needs an additional dose of medication, it can be difficult to administer subsequent doses to a partially sedated child without the risk of aspiration. The most common sedative medication given via the oral route is midazolam. Orally administered fentanyl ("fentanyl lollipop") and ketamine are also used. The rectal route of administration is most useful in infants and toddlers, as older children are often not amenable to this approach. As with oral medications, rectally administered medications can exhibit a wide range of absorption from patient to patient. One advantage of the rectal route is that subsequent doses can be given if the patient is partially sedated. The most commonly administered rectal sedative medication for pediatric patients is methohexital. Thus, the oral and rectal routes of administration are most useful for sedating infants and children, and the medications administered via these routes have a very wide therapeutic window.

Sedative medications in infants and children also can be given via an injection, which has once been a very popular route of administration. Onset is usually more rapid than with oral medications. Today, however, injections are a less and less popular because of the widespread fear of needles in children and the parental expectation of a more child-friendly approach. All of the narcotics as well as ketamine and midazolam can be given via injection. Most practitioners today use injections only in sedating children who are combative or very uncooperative and refuse to take medication orally or allow IV placement.

The transdermal route is in many ways the most attractive approach to the sedation of infants and children. It is painless, easy to use and ideally, removing the medication from the skin would terminate the effect. Unfortunately, the only sedative medications commonly available for transdermal routes in the form of patches are fentanyl and clonidine. The fentanyl patch is more suitable for the treatment of chronic pain than for sedating pediatric patients, and the clonidine patch is more suitable for treating hypertension than for sedating pediatric patients. The current generation of transdermal delivery systems have relatively slow and variable absorption through the skin and come in a limited number of dosages. If transdermal delivery systems are developed for medications such midazolam, which are both reliable and fast-acting, this could prove to be an exciting alternative for sedating pediatric patients.

The intravenous route of administration of sedative medication allows the practitioner to most reliably establish an effective, consistent blood level of sedative medication. The intravenous route allows the titration of small doses of sedating medication or the use of a pump to provide a continuous infusion of sedative medication. It also allows more rapid adjustments if the level of stimulation during the procedure changes. Intravenous access facilitates the reversal of a narcotic or a benzodiazepine overdose by the administration and titration of naloxone or flumazenil. Intravenous access also facilitates resuscitation of the patient with intravenous fluids and medications, if necessary. While not the simplest, the intravenous route is the best and safest approach to providing adequate sedation in pediatric patients while minimizing side effects. Therefore, the first challenge in providing reliable, effective, and safe sedation of the pediatric patient is establishing intravenous access.

Not only is it often more technically difficult to place an IV in infants and children because their veins are smaller, but they are often uncooperative and fearful of IV placement. As a result of this, numerous strategies have evolved to facilitate establishing intravenous access in children. Older children may be cooperative with IV placement, especially if local anesthesia such as lidocaine is used to facilitate IV placement. Infants and children of all ages will benefit from the use of EMLA cream that, when placed 45–60 minutes prior to the sedation, makes IV placement painless and often nontraumatic in children. Alternatively, a pre-sedation medication given orally, such as midazolam, will facilitate IV placement. In children who are uncooperative and unwilling to take a pre-sedation medication orally, IM ketamine is an approach of last resort.

It is important to realize that a highly effective nonpharmacologic adjunct to the initiation of sedation in pediatric patients is parental presence, which sometimes can provide a calming influence during the initiation of sedation or during IV placement. If parental presence is used during the initiation of sedation, the parent(s) must be told in advance what to expect when their infant or child loses consciousness. They must also be told in advance when they must leave the child. Ideally, the parent(s) would then be personally escorted to a waiting area. It is important to have an additional caregiver assigned to escort the parents to the waiting area and to calm and reassure them. It is important to realize that while parental presence can be helpful and calming to the child, in certain situations it can be less than helpful and make the initiation of sedation more difficult. If the parents are extremely anxious and nervous, often this anxiety will be transferred to the child and may make the initiation of sedation more difficult.

Just as parental presence can be helpful during the initiation of sedation, parental presence often can be helpful during the recovery from sedation. Children waking up in a different and strange environment such as the hospital are often disoriented. Parental presence can provide reassurance and be very comforting to the child. Assuming it is logistically possible, parental presence during recovery from sedation should be encouraged.

Remote Locations

If at all possible, care and planning should go into making all locations in which children are sedated as safe and ergonomic as possible for the care and resuscitation of children. Ideally, there should be more than one pipeline source of oxygen mounted on the wall, which would include both a flowmeter for delivering supplemental oxygen via a nasal canula or face mask and a connection appropriate for an anesthesia machine. These would ideally be placed in the room in a location that is both near the head of the patient while the procedure is being performed and allows for the placement of an anesthesia machine. Located with the wall oxygen source should be a wall suction source. If there is only one source of oxygen, alternative oxygen supplies in the form of oxygen tanks need to be immediately available.

Monitors must be placed in a location that allows for easy visual access for the person responsible for monitoring the patient. In locations in which remote monitoring will occur, such as in the MRI scanner, a second set of monitors should be available. Electrical outlets for the multiple monitors should be numerous and placed in appropriate locations so that extension cords are not extensively used and do not become hazards. Ideally, a movable light source should be available to both aid in intravenous cannulation and assist in visually monitoring the patient's color and respiratory efforts. Every effort should be made to design locations in which sedation will occur so that the person administering the sedation and monitoring the patient has quick and easy access to all necessary equipment and supplies.

The ideal location for sedation would also be child-friendly and designed to allow the parents to be present for the initiation of sedation. Recovery facilities should be nearby, precluding the necessity of transporting pediatric patients for long distances or using elevators.

It is important to remember that each sedating location has unique characteristics that can provide unique challenges. Many of the radiology locations such as the CT scanner, interventional radiology, and the cardiac catheterization laboratory use radiation. It is important for the practitioners providing the sedation to protect themselves from excessive radiation by using appropriate lead aprons and remaining as far from the radiation beam, while still being able to effectively monitor and sedate the patient. The MRI suite has unique characteristics in that much of the equipment commonly used may be ferromagnetic and can be inadvertently pulled into the magnet, which can cause serious injury if a patient is within the magnet range. Special MRI-compatible monitors must be used to measure the patient's oxygen saturation, end-tidal CO_2, and blood pressure. Most infusion pumps will need to be placed at a significant distance from the magnet depending on the strength of the magnet and how well shielded the magnet is to ensure that they are not pulled into the magnet and to ensure that the pumps function accurately within the MRI environment.

Drug Selection for Sedating Pediatric Patients

Many practitioners seek one drug that will reliably sedate all pediatric patients at the same dosage for all procedures. Unfortunately, no such magic elixir exists. The practitioner must decide which drug or combination of drugs will most effectively sedate a particular pediatric patient for a particular procedure. This decision must take into account the patient's allergies, prior history with sedative drugs, and particular risk factors. For example, pediatric patients with a history of sleep apnea will be particularly sensitive to narcotic agents. This decision also must take into account the length and nature of the procedure. If the procedure is not painful, such as an MRI scan, the use of narcotics is often not necessary. However, if the procedure is painful, such as a procedure in interventional radiology, it is be difficult to effectively sedate the patient without the use of narcotics or other analgesic agents. Longer procedures require either the use of longer-acting agents or preferably the use of repeat dosages of shorter-acting agents or a continuous infusion to maintain constant blood levels of the drug. In general, drugs that are rapidly acting and rapidly cleared are preferable because they allow a rapid awakening from sedation and a quick recovery and return to baseline. Drugs that have minimal side effects and do not cause significant cardiac or respiratory depression obviously decrease morbidity and mortality.

Chloral Hydrate

Chloral hydrate has been used for many years to provide sedation for painless procedures, as it has no analgesic properties. It has proven particularly useful for diagnostic imaging studies, such as CT scans, MRI scans, and EEGs. Its

TABLE 3. Recommendations for Drug Dosages for Sedation of Pediatric Patients

Drug	Route	Dosage	Time of Onset (min)	Duration of Action (min)
Midazolam	PO	0.5–1.0 mg/kg (max 15 mg)	20–30	60–90
Midazolam	IN, PR	0.2–0.5 mg/kg	10–30	50–75
Midazolam	IM	0.1–0.2 mg/kg	10–15	60–90
Midazolam	IV	0.02–0.1 mg/kg	5–10	30–60
Chloral hydrate	PO	25–100 mg/kg	15–30	60–120
Pentobarbital	PO, PR	2–4 mg/kg (max 100 mg)	20–60	60–240
Pentobarbital	IV	1–2 mg/kg	3–5	20–40
Methohexital	PR	25 mg/kg	10–20	60–75
Fentanyl	IV, IM	0.5–1.0 µg/kg	2–4	30–60
Fentanyl	PO	10–20 µg/kg	10–30	120–240
Meperidine	IV, IM	0.2–0.5 mg/kg	4–8	60–90
Morphine	IV, IM	0.05–0.1 mg/kg	5–10	45–120
Ketamine	IM	3–5 mg/kg	3–6	30–180
Ketamine	IV	0.5–1.0 mg/kg	1–2	15–60
Naloxone	IM	0.1 mg/kg	10–15	60–90
Naloxone	IV	0.1 mg/kg	2–4	30–40
Flumazenil	IV	0.01–0.02 mg/kg	1–2	30–60
Propofol	IV	Initial bolus: 1–2 mg/kg	1–2	5–15
Propofol	IV	Infusion: 50–250 µg/kg/min	–	–

PO, orally; PR, rectally; IM, intramuscularly; IN, intranasally; IV, intravenously.

major advantage is that it can be given orally or rectally and does not require the presence of an IV access. A dose of 50–100 mg/kg often provides sedation for 90–120 minutes. Its limitations include the fact that it only provides sedation and does not provide any analgesia and is inappropriate for any painful or stimulating procedures. It must be given 20–30 minutes prior to the procedure and has a significant failure rate, with infants and children not being adequately sedated despite a second dose. Another disadvantage is that the sedation often persists for hours after the end of the procedure. Significant respiratory depression and/or aspiration can occur with chloral hydrate administration.

Demerol/Phenergan/Thorazine (DPT)

The combination of meperidine (Demerol) at 2 mg/kg, promethazine (Phenergan) at 1 mg/kg, and chlorpromazine (Thorazine) at 1 mg/kg as an intramuscular injection has also been extensively used in the past for the sedation of pediatric patients. As this medication can only be given as an injection and because of its high incidence of complications and its prolonged recovery period, DPT cannot be recommended for the routine sedation of pediatric patients.

Ketamine

Ketamine is another anesthetic drug with a long history of use, which can be administered intramuscularly as an injection, intravenously, orally, or rectally. It produces a dissociative state with analgesia, immobilization, amnesia, and sedation and in high doses can produce anesthesia. While it is generally associated with the maintenance of spontaneous ventilation, it also is associated with increased oral secretions and can result in respiratory depression. The concurrent use of glycopyrrolate can reduce the degree of oral secretions. Unfortunately, ketamine is associated with unpleasant emergence reactions, including hallucinations and nightmares that can persist for several weeks after the procedure. The concurrent use of benzodiazepines reduces, but does not eliminate, these unpleasant side effects.

Barbiturates

Rectal methohexital and intravenous pentobarbital have been extensively used for nonpainful procedures such as radiologic diagnostic imaging. Like chloral hydrate, the barbiturates lack analgesic properties. While pentobarbital also can be given intramuscularly, orally, or rectally, it is most commonly given intravenously because it can be titrated to effect with multiple smaller doses. It also has a relatively rapid onset of action. The disadvantages of both methohexital and pentobarbital are primarily related to the prolonged postprocedural sedation. Pentobarbital can be combined with analgesic agents such as fentanyl, but the risk of respiratory depression and respiratory obstruction increases significantly.

Midazolam

Midazolam is one of the most popular drugs for sedation of pediatric patients. It produces anxiolysis and amnesia in lower doses, and in higher doses produces significant sedation. It is a short-acting benzodiazepine that can be given orally, intranasally, rectally, intramuscularly, or intravenously. It has a very rapid onset of action given intravenously and can be titrated to effect with multiple smaller doses. Its onset of action is slower if given intramuscularly or intranasally and slowest when given rectally and orally. When used orally it can facilitate separation from the parents and intravenous cannulation. It can result in respiratory depression if given in high doses, and narcotics such as fentanyl potentiate its respiratory depressant effects. It should only be used when benzodiazepine antagonist flumazenil is readily available.

Narcotics

Morphine, meperidine, and fentanyl are all narcotics that can be given either intramuscularly or intravenously to provide sedation of pediatric patients. Fentanyl is shorter-acting than morphine and meperidine with a faster onset and shorter duration of action, and its use is not associated with histamine release. Because of these factors and the ability to titrate small doses intravenously, it is rapidly becoming the most common narcotic used for pediatric sedation. Morphine and meperidine should be reserved for longer, painful procedures in which one anticipates significant postprocedural pain. Fentanyl also can be administered transdermally via a fentanyl patch and orally via a fentanyl "lollipop." The transdermal route results in a slower absorption than the intravenous route, precluding its routine use for sedation. Administering fentanyl orally is associated with a high rate of emesis. Like all of the narcotics, fentanyl is associated with side effects, incuding respiratory depression that can be profound, nausea and vomiting, and pruritus. Fentanyl, morphine, and meperidine should only be used when naloxone is readily available and when both personnel and equipment to support the airway are readily available. Newer shorter-acting narcotics such as remifentanil are currently available. They are so short-acting that they must be administered by an infusion for all but the briefest procedures. Remifentanil's potency and ability to produce profound respiratory and cardiac depression preclude its use for routine sedation of pediatric patients by nonanesthesiologists.

Propofol

Propofol is an intravenous agent that can produce excellent sedation and immobility, is very rapidly metabolized, and has a very short duration of action. It is most commonly given via an infusion. Its disadvantages include the fact that it can be painful when injected and is relatively expensive. It produces minimal analgesia, but can produce profound respiratory and cardiac depression. Its major advantages are that it produces virtually no side effects and is very rapidly cleared, allowing a return to preprocedural status often in less than 30 minutes. Because of its profound respiratory and cardiac depressant effects and because in higher doses it produces general anesthesia, its use is limited to anesthesiologists.

Drug Dosage Recommendations

There is no single dosage or range of dosages that is both safe and effective in every patient. The safest approach is to titrate to effect using smaller dosages and administer subsequent doses on an as-needed basis, taking into account the time of peak onset of the drug being used (Table 3). Knowing that fentanyl's time of peak onset is shorter than morphine's, for example, allows the practitioner to administer a subsequent dose of fentanyl sooner than a subsequent dose of morphine. In some pediatric patients, the doses of medication required will exceed the recommendations, such as patients who have been taking narcotic pain medications. Their tolerance to these drugs is higher and they require larger and more frequent doses of narcotics for sedation. In some other patients it is prudent to start with a lower than recommended dose of medication for sedation. When administering intravenous doses of sedative medication it is always easier to give an additional dose than to deal with the consequences of oversedation. Pediatric patients in whom one should consider smaller doses include those who are obese, have obstructive sleep apnea, and even those whose parents report night-time snoring. Patients with decreased hepatic or renal function also should have the dosages of sedative medications appropriately reduced. It is also important to consider reducing the doses of a particular sedative medication if a combination of sedative drugs is going to be used.

References

1. American Academy of Pediatrics Committee on Drugs: Guidelines for Monitoring and Management of Pediatric Patients during and after Sedation for Diagnostic and Therapeutic Procedures. Pediatrics 89:1110–1115, 1992.
2. American Society of Anesthesiologists Professional Information, Continuum of Depth of Sedation, Definition of General Anesthesia and Levels of Sedation/Analgesia. (http://www.asahq.org/Standards/20.htm) Approved October 13, 1999.
3. Cote CJ: Sedation for the pediatric patient: A review. Pediatr Clin North Am 41:31–58, 1994.
4. Cote CJ, Notterman DA, Karl HW, et al: Adverse sedation events in pediatrics: A critical incident analysis of contributing factors. Pediatrics 105:805–814, 2000.
5. Krauss B, Green SM: Sedation and analgesia for procedures in children. New Engl J Med 342:938–945, 2000
6. Practice Guidelines for Sedation and Analgesia by Non-Anesthsiologists: A Report by the American Society of Anesthesiologists Task Force on Sedation and Analgesia by Non-Anesthesiologists. Anesthesiology 84:459–471, 1996.

7. Siberry GK (ed): The Harriet Lane Handbook, 15th ed. St. Louis, Mosby, 2000.
8. Warner MA, Caplan RA, Epstein BS, et al: Practice guidelines for preoperative fasting and the use of pharmacologic agents to reduce the risk of pulmonary aspiration: Application to healthy patients undergoing elective procedures. Anesthesiology 90:896–905, 1999.

8

Conscious Sedation in the Elderly

Linda L. Liu, M.D.

The American population is aging. Twenty-five million people are now over the age of 65, and 2.7 million are over the age of 85. Projected estimates by the U.S. Census Bureau for the year 2030 indicate that one in five persons in the U.S. (approximately 35 million people) will be older than age 65, and 1 in 4 of the elderly will be older than age 85.[1] These individuals 65 years of age or older will account for one-third of the surgical procedures performed annually, and use one-third of all health care expenditures.

The use of conscious sedation has become very common and estimates are that more and more cases may be performed outside of the operating room. The procedures performed can range from inpatient to outpatient as well as therapeutic to diagnostic to surgical. Patient demand has influenced part of this trend. Surveys have shown that the elderly actually prefer more ambulatory settings for surgical procedures.[14] Pressure from the insurance companies is the second reason for this current trend. For instance, Medicare has started favoring more outpatient protocols for certain procedures.

Caution must be used in providing sedation for the elderly. They are a diverse population, and no two people age in the same way. The aging diminishes organ function and limits physiologic reserves. Sedation should be individualized based on the planned procedure and the patient's specific needs. This chapter defines basic principles important to sedation of the elderly by examining the physiologic changes associated with aging and reviewing the pharmacokinetics and pharmacodynamics of commonly used drugs that are altered with advancing age.

Physiologic Changes Associated with Aging

Under normal conditions, the physiologic changes that occur with aging are not readily evident and lead to minimal functional impairment. But with the

TABLE 1. Changes Associated with Aging

Body Composition
- ↓ lean body mass
- ↑ body fat
- ↓ total body water

Cardiovascular System
- ↓ elasticity (left ventricular hypertrophy)
- ↓ cardiac output
- ↓ beta-adrenergic responsiveness
- ↑ incidence of ischemic heart disease

Respiratory System
- ↓ chest wall compliance
- ↑ lung compliance
- ↓ alveolar gas exchange surface
- ↑ closing capacity and residual volume
- ↓ upper airway reflexes
- ↓ response to hypoxia and hypercarbia

Thermoregulation
- ↓ temperature regulation
- ↓ vasoconstriction and shivering

Hepatic System
- ↓ hepatic mass
- ↓ liver blood flow
- ↓ protein synthesis (albumin)
- ↓ drug clearance

Renal System
- ↓ renal mass
- ↓ renal blood flow
- ↓ ability to concentrate urine and conserve free water
- ↓ ability to secrete acid and conserve sodium

Central Nervous System
- ↓ neurons and cerebral mass
- ↓ neurotransmitters
- ↓ sensory input
- ↑ sensitivity to anesthetics
- ↑ incidence of postoperative delirium

↑, increased; ↓, decreased.

onset of a stressful situation like illness or surgery, the elderly may then display diminished reserve capacity and be more prone to complications. Table 1 summarizes the changes associated with aging that are reviewed in this chapter.

Body Composition

There are three changes in body composition associated with aging. These include a loss of skeletal muscle (decreased lean body mass), increased body fat, and decreased total body water. All these changes happen to a greater degree in women. The smaller central compartment due to decreased total body water can result in a higher peak concentration following boluses or rapid infusions. In other words, the injection of anesthetic drugs will be dispersed in an initially smaller blood volume. The increased body fat leads to an increased lipid storage site and a larger compartment for lipid-soluble drugs. This could potentially result in an increased total volume of distribution and a longer duration of drug effect. For the elderly population, clinically this means smaller bolus doses and longer intervals between doses.

Cardiovascular System

With aging, there is loss of elasticity in the large arteries, which leads to increased systolic pressure and increased afterload for the left ventricle. Over time, increased workload on the ventricle results in left ventricular hypertrophy. Due to the hypertrophy, elderly patients require higher filling pressures in order to maintain stroke volume and cardiac output. For the elderly, cardiac output is maintained by increasing end-diastolic volume during exercise.[23] Cardiac output declines by 1% per year after the age of 50 and the maximal heart rate is markedly decreased due to decreased responsiveness to beta-adrenergic agonists.[16]

The decreased elasticity also contributes to higher incidences of hypertension and ischemic heart disease. The frequency of coronary artery disease is estimated to exceed 80% in octogenarians.[17] Forty percent of 80-year-olds have symptomatic cardiac disease,[35] and as many as 10% may have congestive heart failure.[11]

The implications for sedative drugs are multifold. The elderly heart will be more sensitive to the decrease in cardiac output caused by these drugs,[32] which may lead to increased hypotension after administration. The changes noted above all lead to a decrease in the available reserve should something go wrong. The elderly patients need special attention to hemodynamic monitoring in order to assure that myocardial oxygen demand does not exceed supply.

Respiratory System

Aging leads to a decline in the elasticity of the chest wall, a weakening of the muscles of respirations, and a decrease in alveolar gas exchange surface.[24] These changes manifest as air trapping, increased closing capacity, and gas exchange problems. Alveolar surface area decreases from 75 m² to about 60 m² at age 70.[34] The mean PaO_2 declines with age, dropping to about 75 ± 5 mmHg at age 75. Beyond this age, the PaO_2 decline plateaus and the PaO_2 remains around 75 mmHg. The elderly may not even tolerate small doses of sedatives because they have significantly decreased ventilatory responses to hypercapnia and hypoxia.[15] A small change in oxygen level could result in significant hypoxemia, so supplemental oxygen is necessary during sedation procedures.

The elderly may also have a decrease in upper airway reflex sensitivity, possibly owing to a reduction in the nerve ending of the irritant receptor.[5] This results in an earlier loss of protective reflexes such as coughing and swallowing and the potential for aspiration with minimal to no sedation. This means more attention needs to be given to assessing the level of consciousness in the elderly during conscious sedation procedures.

Hepatic System

Liver blood flow is decreased as a result of lower cardiac output, and hepatic protein synthesis is decreased as well.[36] Some studies report that as much as a 30% decrease in drug metabolism can occur with aging. The overall effect is to decrease the clearance of sedative drugs and reduce the maintenance dose that is required for sedation in the elderly. Drugs that are not metabolized via the liver, such as remifentanil, are not affected by this decrement in liver function.

Renal System

As one ages, the decrease in cardiac output leads to a drop in renal blood flow and the glomerular filtration rate (GFR). The GFR is estimated to decrease by 6–8% per decade of life.[21] Even in an elderly patient with a normal creatinine, the creatinine clearance can be one-half that of normal. The effect of this decline in renal function is an increase in the elimination half-life of drugs cleared by the kidneys. Dosing intervals for drugs excreted by the kidney will need to be lengthened.

Other renal functions such as the ability to concentrate urine and conserve free water as well as the ability to secrete an acid load and conserve sodium are decreased.[4] This could predispose the elderly patient after prolonged fasting to dehydration, hemodynamic instability, and alterations in electrolytes.

Central Nervous System

The effects of aging are multifold on the brain. There is selective loss of cerebral and cerebellar cortical neurons in the thalamus, locus ceruleus, and basal ganglia. By age 80, there is a 30% decrease in brain mass and a decreased number of serotonin, acetylcholine, and dopamine receptors.[20] There is also a concurrent decrease in cerebral blood flow and oxygen consumption. Memory and reasoning performance decline and there are increased thresholds for vision, hearing, touch, joint position sense, smell, and peripheral pain and temperature. Components listed above may lead to the high incidence of postoperative delirium observed in the elderly.[19] Overall, the elderly tend to have lower anesthetic requirements,[22] be more sensitive to sedatives, and have a prolonged recovery.

The elderly also have more vascular narrowing of the carotid arteries. Patients older than 74 years have an average of 2 carotid plaques per patient, 20.5% of whom have 3 or more plaques.[30] Care should be taken to maintain pre-operative cerebral blood flow and oxygen delivery since aging changes make the elderly brain more susceptible to ischemia.

Thermoregulation

Due to the altered responses to changes in body temperature, elderly patients are unable to regulate body temperature like younger patients. Their response to hypothermia is delayed and shivering does not occur until a much lower temperature.[33] The inability to vasoconstrict and reduce skin blood flow makes heat loss in a cold environment much greater. Even taking the decreased shivering into account, recovery from hypothermia is delayed in the elderly due to their lower metabolic rate, which produces less heat. The hypothermia may also last longer and it can exacerbate the decreased clearance of drugs already present in the elderly. Extra attention should be taken during conscious sedation procedures even if they are relatively short. Conservative measures include warming the procedure room and keeping the patient covered with blankets for as long as possible. Using warmed solutions for prepping and intravenous fluids will also help decrease the loss of temperature. Forced-air blankets can be very helpful for longer procedures.

Effects of Aging on Common Sedative Drugs

To understand how the physiologic changes that occur with aging affect specific drug actions, a few terms must first be defines. Pharmacokinetics is the study of drug absorption, distribution, metabolism, and elimination. Three of the four are affected by aging, but the first, drug absorption, is often unchanged. Drug distribution is affected by the volume of distribution, which is decreased in the elderly due to decreased total body water. Metabolism and elimination are both decreased due to decreased function of the renal and hepatic systems. This increase in elimination half-life can make the elderly more susceptible to adverse drug reactions. Pharmacodynamics is the effect that the drug has on the body, and it appears that end-organ sensitivity may change with age.[28] The elderly are often more sensitive to various drugs when compared to a younger cohort.

The following section reviews several common drugs used in conscious sedation from a pharmacokinetic and pharmacodynamic standpoint. Unfortunately, much of the data are often inconsistent. Problems in comparing studies involved wide interindividual variations (gender and race) and confounding variables such as other metabolic pathways and other extrinsic factors (hormones, alcohol, and tobacco). Although the authors may not all agree on the exact reason why the elderly need less sedative drugs, they all eventually agree that this phenomenon does occur.

Drugs such as thiopental, propofol, and remifentanil have been included since they are commonly used in anesthesia. They should be used with caution or avoided all together by personnel not trained in airway management. They tend to have a rapid onset of action and can quickly lead to unconsciousness, loss of airway reflexes, and apnea.

Thiopental

Thiopental, a barbiturate and commonly used drug in anesthesia, has been extensively studied from a pharmacokinetic and pharmacodynamic standpoint. Early studies using electroencephalography (EEG) proved that the increased sensitivity of elderly patients to this drug was not due to increased brain sensitivity, but rather a decreased volume of distribution.[10] For any equal dose of drug, the elderly had a higher drug level in the bloodstream. The models predict that a 15% reduction of thiopental dose would be necessary for the induction of anesthesia in a healthy 80-year-old compared with a 20-year-old due to the smaller volume of distribution. As the first compartment equilibrates with the larger fat compartment, the differences in infusion rates to maintain anesthesia become equal after about 90 minutes.[29] When the infusion is discontinued, recovery from thiopental is slow, but the effect of age is negligible (i.e., the recovery is equally slow for the young and the old).

Propofol

Propofol, a lipid-soluble sedative hypnotic that produces rapid induction of anesthesia, is associated with minimal residual sedative effects upon awakening. Because of its rapidity of onset and offset, this drug is popular among anesthesiologists for anesthesia as well as conscious sedation cases. From pharmacokinetic studies, it appeared that the elderly had a reduced clearance and a smaller volume of distribution. Like thiopental, elderly patients required only 80–90% of the induction dose used on younger patients if only pharmacokinetics were considered. Unfortunately, this was at odds with clinical observation that anesthesia could be induced with only 1 mg/kg of propofol in the elderly. To resolve the conflict, the pharmacodynamics of propofol had to be investigated. It became apparent that the brain becomes more sensitive to propofol with aging when

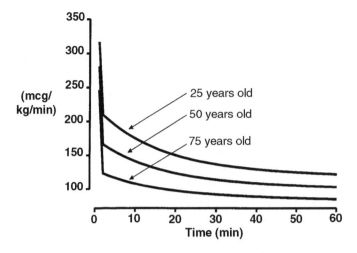

Figure 1. Age-adjusted infusions of propofol for general anesthesia based on pharmacokinetic and pharmacodynamic data. (From Schafer SL: The pharmacology of anesthetic drugs in elderly patients. Anesthesiol Clin North Am 18:1–29, 2000, with permission.)

EEG is used to follow the onset of drug effect.[25] The effect is almost 30% more sensitive in the elderly. Figure 1 illustrates the decrease in dosing that would be necessary based on known pharmacokinetic and pharmacodynamic models. It is important to note that these figures are based on drug dose required for adequate anesthesia. Infusion for conscious sedation would have to be drastically reduced from these values, and titrated to effect.

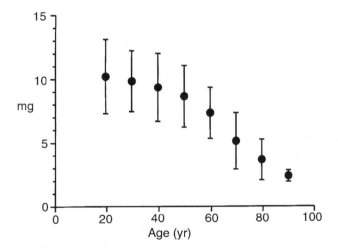

Figure 2. Influence of age on the dose of midazolam required for endoscopy. (From Bell GD, Spickett GP, Reeve PA, et al: Intravenous midazolam for upper gastrointestinal endoscopy: A study of 800 consecutive cases relating dose to age and sex of patient. Br J Clin Pharmacol 23:241–243, 1987, with permission.)

Midazolam

Midazolam is a short-acting benzodiazepine that is commonly used for anesthesia and conscious sedation. It is often used as a premedication to induce anxiolysis, sedation and amnesia. In a study of 800 patients undergoing endoscopy, the total dose of midazolam ranged from an average of 10 mg in 20-year-olds down to an average of 2–3 mg in 80–90-year-olds.[2] Figure 2 shows the data graphically.

From the pharmacokinetic data, it appears that the clearance, volume of distribution, and elimination half-life of midazolam range from no difference to only a modest 25% change as compared with younger patients. Using EEG as a measure of sedative hypnotic effect, the elderly again show much more sensitivity to the sedative effects of this drug. It is this pharmocodynamic effect that explains the almost 50–75% reduction in dose that is required in the elderly. In a recent study involving 90 geriatric patients undergoing transuretheral procedures, an oxygen saturation (SPO_2) of less than 94% was obtained in 90% (27 patients) of the patients who received 2 mg midazolam intravenously, and 42% (12 patients) of the patients who received only 0.5 mg midazolam. Although the groups showed no difference from placebo on mental status testing postoperatively, the times to recovery room discharge were significantly longer in both midazolam groups.[6]

Diazepam

Like midazolam, diazepam has properties of amnesia, anxiolysis, and sedation that are valuable in conscious sedation, but it is much slower in onset and has a markedly longer half-life. Diazepam is less readily used in anesthesia due to its long duration of action. When used properly, its slower onset of action makes oversedation and loss of airway reflexes less likely than with propofol. Its low cost also makes the drug attractive.

Multiple studies found that the volume of distribution is increased with diazepam and clearance is decreased. Elimination half-life studies show a prolongation from 20 hours at age 20 to 90 hours at age 80.[12,13] Like all the benzodiazepines, there is increased sensitivity to this drug in the elderly, necessitating marked decrease in initial dose as well as a longer interval between repeat dosing. Diazepam also has an active metabolite (desmethyldiazepam). This drug is probably not the drug of choice to be using in the elderly with its associated negative pharmacokinetic and pharmacodynamic changes.

The studies seem to suggest that benzodiazepines that are biotransformed by microsomal oxidation (diazepam, midazolam) are associated with impaired clearance, while benzodiazepines metabolised mainly by glucuronide conjugation (lorazepam) are less impaired with aging.[8] For all drugs in this class there are pharmacodynamic changes, making the elderly much more sensitive to their effects. In summary, adjustments in dosing must be considered when providing conscious sedation with any benzodiazepine in the elderly.

Fentanyl

Fentanyl has been the most popular narcotic among anesthesiologists due to its rapid onset of action, short duration, and low cost. The drug has been studied extensively in the elderly and EEG has been used to measure its pharmacodynamic effects. Scott et al. were unable to find any effect of age on the pharmacokinetics of fentanyl.[26] What they did find was a 50% decrease in the plasma concentration required for EEG depression from the young (age 20) to the elderly (age 85). These results imply that elderly patients require only half the dose of fentanyl that younger patients require due to pharmacodynamic changes. Because pharmacokinetics are not greatly altered, when dosed appropriately, the dissipation of drug effect should be the same in the two age groups.

Remifentanil

Remifentanil is a relatively new narcotic that is ultrashort-acting and metabolized by nonspecific tissue and plasma esterases. The volume of distribution of remifentanil decreases about 20%, the clearance decreases by 30%, and the elimination half-life increases in the elderly. Like fentanyl, remifentanil appears to be twice as effective in the elderly based on data from EEG depression.[18]

Figure 3 shows that based on the above data, the elderly need only half the bolus dose used in younger patients, and one third the infusion rate due to the increased sensitivity and decreased clearance in the elderly. If the dose is appropriately reduced, recovery from remifentanil in the elderly is as rapid as in the younger population.

Morphine

Morphine is a longer-acting narcotic that has a slower onset time than fentanyl and remifentanil. Unlike the other narcotics, it does have metabolites that contribute some activity and may increase adverse effects. Although the volume of distribution is relatively unchanged, the clearance of morphine is markedly decreased in the elderly.[27] It appears that like the other drugs, the initial bolus and subsequent dosing intervals should be adjusted for the elderly.

Meperidine

Meperidine, introduced in the 1940s, has been used by many nonanesthesiologists to provide conscious sedation. Its use by anesthesiologists is more limited to the treatment of postoperative shivering as there are other drugs with faster onsets and better side effect profiles. When studied as a single intravenous dose for premedication, meperidine given to older patients had a lower plasma

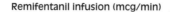

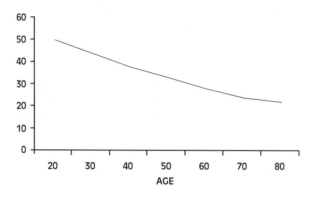

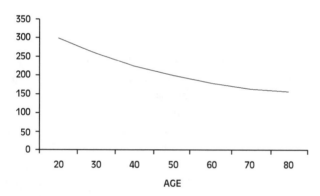

Figure 3. Age-adjusted infusions of remifentanil based on pharmacokinetic and pharmacodynamic data. (Modified from Minto CF, Schnider TW, Shafer SL: The influence of age and gender on the pharmacokinetics and pharmacodynamics of remifentanil: II. Model application. Anesthesiology 86:24–33, 1997.)

clearance and longer elimination half-life. The volume of distribution was similar between the two groups.

Of note, normeperidine, an active metabolite, reached its peak concentration later in the elderly, and was still present longer (up to 30 hours).[9] Since there are many other available choices of narcotics, meperidine should probably not be used in the elderly.

Preoperative Assessment

It appears from multiple studies that the complication rate is probably more a function of concurrent diseases than due to age alone.[3] Therefore, associated medical problems must be illicited prior to the start of conscious sedation so that the depth and type of sedation administered can be determined. Other medications should be listed due to an increased incidence of adverse drug interactions in the elderly. Basically, a thorough history and physical examination should be performed and documented in the chart prior to the start of the case. If the patient appears to be too ill for the department to handle, alternate arrangements should be made for access to better monitoring and/or anesthesia care.

The overall risk of perioperative complications in the elderly is increased, but still relatively low. Tiret et al. found a 0.5% rate of complications in patients older than 80 years of age undergoing anesthesia.[31] Procedures performed under conscious sedation are less invasive and should have even lower anticipated complications if care is used to obtain a thorough history; drugs are dosed appropriately, and homeostasis is maintained.

Summary

The elderly pose specific challenges for conscious sedation due to alterations in the cardiovascular, pulmonary, neurologic, and hepatorenal systems. They tend to have a larger variability in drug response along with decreased requirements for most anesthetic drugs and increased redosing intervals. Standard dosages based on weight should be avoided and slower administration with more time allowance for peak effect can often achieve good sedation with a lower total dose.

In the future, bispectral index monitoring (BIS) may be routinely used to help monitor the level of sedation. This may allow better titration of sedatives and allow less drug use.[7] These monitors are currently being used in the operating room to help with titration of general anesthesia. For now, sedation in the elderly patient should be individualized based on the patient's needs and the needs of the procedure. For conscious sedation to be administered safely to the elderly population, meticulous attention must be paid to monitoring, and the administration of sedatives must be given cautiously and titrated to clinical effect.

References

1. http://www.census.gov/population/nation/intfile2-1.txt, 1998.
2. Bell GD, Spickett GP, Reeve PA, et al: Intravenous midazolam for upper gastrointestinal endoscopy: A study of 800 consecutive cases relating dose to age and sex of patient. Br J Clin Pharmacol 23:241–243, 1987.
3. Dunlop WE, Rosenblood L, Lawrason L, et al: Effects of age and severity of illness on outcome and length of stay in geriatric surgical patients. Am J Surg 165:577–580, 1993.
4. Epstein M: Aging and the kidney. J Am Soc Nephrol 7:1106–1122, 1996.

5. Erskine RJ, Murphy PJ, Langton JA, et al: Effect of age on the sensitivity of upper airway reflexes. Br J Anaesth 70:574–575, 1993.

6. Fredman B, Lahav M, Zohar E, et al: The effect of midazolam premedication on mental and psychomotor recovery in geriatric patients undergoing brief surgical procedures. Anesth Analg 89:1161–1166, 1999.

7. Glass PS, Bloom M, Kearse L, et al: Bispectral analysis measures sedation and memory effects of propofol, midazolam, isoflurane, and alfentanil in healthy volunteers. Anesthesiology 86:836–847, 1997.

8. Greenblatt DJ, Harmatz JS, Shader RI: Clinical pharmacokinetics of anxiolytics and hypnotics in the elderly. Therapeutic considerations (Part II). Clin Pharmacokinetics 21:262–273, 1991.

9. Holmberg L, Odar-Cederlöf I, Boréus LO, et al: Comparative disposition of pethidine and norpethidine in old and young patients. Eur J Clin Pharmacol 22:175–179, 1982.

10. Homer TD, Stanski DR: The effect of increasing age on thiopental disposition and anesthetic requirement. Anesthesiology 62:714–724, 1985.

11. Kannel WB, Belanger AJ: Epidemiology of heart failure. Am Heart J 121:951, 1991.

12. Klotz U: Pathophysiological and disease-induced changes in drug distribution volume: pharmacokinetic implications. Clin Pharmacokinetics 1:204–218, 1976.

13. Klotz U, Avant GR, Hoyumpa A, et al: The effects of age and liver disease on the disposition and elimination of diazepam in adult man. J Clin Invest 55:347–359, 1975.

14. Koska MT: Ambulatory surgery gets high marks from the elderly. Hospitals 64:55, 1990.

15. Kronenberg R, Drage C: Attenuation of the ventilatory and heart rate responses to hypozia and hypercarbia with aging in normal men. J Clin Invest 52:1812, 1973.

16. Lakatta E: Diminished beta-adrenergic modulation of cardiovascular function in advanced age. Cardiol Clin 4:185, 1986.

17. Mangano DT: Perioperative cardiac morbidity. Anesthesiology 72:153–184, 1990.

18. Minto CF, Schnider TW, Egan TD, et al: Influence of age and gender on the pharmacokinetics and pharmacodynamics of remifentanil. I. Model development. Anesthesiology 86:10–23, 1997.

19. Moller J, Cluitmans P, Rasmussen L, et al: Long-term postoperative cognitive dysfunction in the elderly: ISPPOCD1 study. Lancet 351:857–861, 1998.

20. Muravchick S: The physiologic and pharmacologic implications of aging. ASA Annual Refresher Course Lectures, p 275, 1986.

21. Muravchick S: Anaesthesia for the aging patient. Can J Anaesth 40:R63–73, 1993.

22. Quasha A, Eger E, Tinker J: Determination and applications of MAC. Anesthesiology 53:315–334, 1980.

23. Rodeheffer R, Gerstenblith G, Becker L, et al: Exercise cardiac output is maintained with advancing age in healthy human subjects: Cardiac dilatation and increased stroke volume compensate for a diminished heart rate. Circulation 69:203–213, 1984.

24. Ross B: Aging and the respiratory system. In Rooke G (ed): Syllabus on Geriatric Anesthesiology. The Committee on Geriatric Anesthesia, March 2000, pp 7–11.

25. Schnider TW, Minto CF, Shafer SL, et al: The influence of age on propofol pharmacodynamics. Anesthesiology 90:1502–1516, 1999.

26. Scott JC, Stanski DR: Decreased fentanyl and alfentanil dose requirements with age: A simultaneous pharmacokinetic and pharmacodynamic evaluation. J Pharmacol Exp Therapeutics 240:159–166, 1987.

27. Sear JW, Hand CW, Moore RA, et al: Studies on morphine disposition: Influence of general anaesthesia on plasma concentrations of morphine and its metabolites. Br J Anaesth 62:22–27, 1989.

28. Shafer S: The pharmacology of anesthetic drugs in elderly patients. Anesth Clin North Am 18:1–29, 2000.

29. Stanski DR, Maitre PO: Population pharmacokinetics and pharmacodynamics of thiopental: The effect of age revisited. Anesthesiology 72:412–422, 1990.

30. Streifler JY, Eliasziw M, Fox AJ, et al: Angiographic detection of carotid plaque ulceration. Comparison with surgical observations in a multicenter study: North American Symptomatic Carotid Endarterectomy Trial. Stroke 25:1130–1132, 1994.

31. Tiret L, Desmonts JM, Hatton F, et al: Complications associated with anaesthesia—a prospective survey in France. Can Anaesth Soc J 33:336–344, 1986.

32. Tokics L, Brismar B, Hedenstierna G: Halothane-relaxant anaesthesia in elderly patients. Acta Anaesth Scand 29:303–308, 1985.

33. Vassilieff N, Rosencher N, Sessler DI, et al: Shivering threshold during spinal anesthesia is reduced in elderly patients. Anesthesiology 83:1162–1166, 1995.

34. Wahba W: Influence of aging on lung function: Clinical significance of changes from age 20. Anesth Analg 62:764–776, 1983.

35. Wei J, Gersh B: Heart disease in the elderly. Curr Probl Cardiol 12:1–65, 1987.

36. Wynne HA, Cope LH, Mutch E, et al: The effect of age upon liver volume and apparent liver blood flow in healthy man. Hepatology 9:297–301, 1989.

9

Conscious Sedation for Endoscopy

Susan M. Ryan, Ph.D., M.D.

Endoscopic procedures provide valuable diagnostic information and therapeutic treatments while having the added benefit of remaining minimally invasive of the gastrointestinal tract. However minimal the intrusion, patients are often anxious and procedures such as colonoscopy and gastroscopy can be uncomfortable or painful. Sedation is often provided for the comfort of the patient and facilitation of the procedure. However, there is controversy regarding the best sedative regimen and the appropriate management and level of monitoring.

Cardiopulmonary complications account for greater than 50% of the total serious complications from endoscopy, and sedation practices have been implicated as a contributing factor. The Food and Drug Administration and the American Society for Gastrointestinal Endoscopy jointly reviewed 21,011 procedures retrospectively in 1991. Cardiorespiratory complications occurred in 5.4 per 1000 procedures with a death rate of 0.3 per 1000.[3] Complications were more likely when narcotics were used in combination with benzodiazepines, or when the endoscopic procedure was an emergency. In 1995, the British Society of Gastroenterology prospectively evaluated 14,149 gastroscopies in two regions of England, including a 30-day follow-up period.[33] They reported a lower rate of cardiopulmonary complication at 2 per 1000. The overall death rate was 0.5 per 1000, with eight deaths from probable aspiration pneumonia, three deaths from pulmonary embolism, and 14 deaths from myocardial infarction. There are multiple differences in these studies, which may account for their differing rates of complications. However, both studies point out that serious complications do occur; in addition, some of their findings suggest that our patient evaluation and selection, sedation, and monitoring practices may help prevent complications. Due in part to these studies, the American Society of Anesthesiologists (ASA) formed an ad hoc committee between 1993 and 1995 to evaluate the issues involved with nonanesthesiologists from a number of fields providing sedation and analgesia. Practice guidelines for sedation and analgesia delivered by nonanesthesiologists were formulated which can apply to gastroenterology as well as other fields such as cardiology.[1] These guidelines form the basis of the following discussion of current practice, sedative and analgesic agents, and a rational strategy for use of conscious sedation in endoscopy.

Is Conscious Sedation for Endoscopy Necessary?

To answer this question, the goals of endoscopy and those of conscious sedation need to be clear in the practitioner's mind. Endoscopic procedures examine and treat different locations in the gastrointestinal tract with the common goals of viewing pathology, taking biopsies for diagnosis, and, in some cases, providing treatment. All of these goals require good patient compliance. Excessive patient movement may prevent an adequate examination, and patient discomfort may force the endoscopist to prematurely terminate an examination. From the endoscopist's perspective, patient cooperation is a major reason to provide sedation. From the viewpoint of the patient, skillful sedation can provide anxiolysis, reduction of discomfort (analgesia), and sometimes amnesia. Therefore, the overall goal of conscious sedation is to safely provide maximum patient cooperation with minimum anxiety and discomfort.

It may seem obvious that conscious sedation is an important adjunct in endoscopic procedures; however, the issue is far from being completely resolved. Most endoscopists are in agreement that the more painful procedures such as percutaneous gastrostomy and esophageal dilation should be performed under sedation and analgesia or general anesthesia. However, for esophagogastroduodenoscopy (EGD), sigmoidoscopy, and colonoscopy, practice and patient expectations differ dramatically throughout the world. Eighty percent of colonoscopies in France are performed under general anesthesia,[21] while absolutely no sedation is provided for most colonoscopy procedures in Germany[14] and Finland.[35] This does not necessarily imply that the patients were uncomfortable in the latter two countries. In Germany, a prospective study examined 2500 patients undergoing colonoscopy.[14] Sedation (midazolam) or analgesia was provided only as needed after initiation of the examination. Ninety-five percent of patients required no medication with complete examinations obtained in greater than 95% of the patients. However, patients were not questioned about comfort afterward. Also, patients have certain expectations prior to the procedure, and they may not expect sedation. Preprocedure expectations and cultural differences may lead to radically differing levels of perceived discomfort from country to country.

In the United States, patients generally expect and receive conscious sedation for most endoscopic procedures. Colonoscopy, more so than upper endoscopy, is widely perceived as painful by patients. Rex et al.[34] attempted to recruit 250 patients into a prospective, randomized trial of sedation versus "sedation as needed" for colonoscopy. Of 250 patients, 163 refused to participate and requested sedation. Seven percent requested not to be sedated, and 27% accepted to be randomized. Ninety-four percent of the "sedation-as-needed" patients completed the study without any sedation. By questionnaire and by endoscopist assessment, they did have more discomfort than their sedated counterparts. All agreed, however, that they would return to the same endoscopist for future procedures.

Upper endoscopy (EGD), even more than colonoscopy, is provided without sedation in a number of countries throughout Asia, Latin America, and Europe. Gagging and discomfort have been reported with the standard-sized endoscopes. Recently, smaller endoscopes have been developed for the purpose of allowing unsedated EGD. Sorbi et al.[41] from the Mayo Clinic compared examinations with conventionally sized endoscopes (c-EGD) to those with small-caliber (6 mm) endoscopes (sc-EGD). They were able to establish feasibility, acceptability, and accuracy of unsedated sc-EGD. Compared with sedated c-EGD (standard-sized), both sedated and unsedated sc-EGD were technically feasible with 96% and 97% accuracy, respectively. On an acceptability scale ranging from 1 (most acceptable) to 10 (least acceptable), overall acceptability was excellent with a median of 1 for sedated c-EGD and 2 for unsedated sc-EGD. None of the 90 patients experienced complications. Ninety-eight percent of the patients undergoing unsedated sc-EGD expressed willingness to undergo the same procedure again.

There are large advantages to foregoing sedation when the unsedated procedure is feasible, acceptable, and accurate. Cardiopulmonary complications related to sedation can be avoided, costs will be lower, recovery times will be shorter, and simple screening procedures could be done in the office instead of the endoscopy suite. The small-caliber endoscope does not have the biopsy or treatment capabilities of the larger endoscopes; however, future improvements in the small-caliber endoscopes can be anticipated. In terms of patient comfort, unsedated small-caliber endoscopy appears to be very well tolerated by most patients. It is less clear that this is true for procedures with standard-sized endoscopes.

Overall, it is clear that patient expectation as well as standard practice in a region will dictate use and extent of sedation. Studies show that some number of patients may not need sedation, and that some are motivated to proceed without it. Endoscopy without sedation or with sedation on an as-needed basis should be offered to appropriate patients as alternatives.

Sedative and Analgesic Agents

Conscious sedation is given to alleviate anxiety and discomfort, thereby improving patient tolerance and improving examination conditions for the endoscopist. Numerous agents have been used to sedate patients for endoscopic procedures. No one regimen reported in the literature appears to be clearly preferred by endoscopists. However, it is important that practitioners examine their goals so that rational sedation strategies may be developed. The approach can be simplified by selecting agents for the alleviation of either anxiety or pain. Secondary considerations of an agent indications, contraindications, side effects, and interactions permits the conscious sedation regimen to be tailored to the individual patient.

Anxiolytics

Most patients who undergo endoscopy are mildly anxious prior to the procedure. This anxiety can easily escalate. Benzodiazepines such as diazepam, lorazepam and midazolam are extremely useful for anxiolysis and mild sedation and are the most frequently used class of medication for upper and lower endoscopy. For upper endoscopy, benzodiazepines are often used alone. Intravenous midazolam, diazepam, and lorazepam have a very short time to onset of sedation and remain clinically effective for the duration of most endoscopic procedures. When first introduced, midazolam was thought to have a lower potency ratio to diazepam, which led to a number of patients being relatively overdosed. With improved understanding of proper dosing, midazolam has become an effective short-acting anxiolytic gaining widespread use.

It is important to understand the limitations of benzodiazepines:

1. They do not have analgesic properties, meaning that pain and discomfort will not be alleviated.

2. Midazolam and lorazepam in particular often provide good anterograde amnesia. This is desirable for someone who does not want to remember the procedure. However, this effect can be magnified in patients taking protease inhibitors. Multiple patients have reported extreme forgetfulness for several days after having received small doses of benzodiazepines (personal communications to author). One patient reported losing objects in his apartment for three days. This could be of great significance if patients forget when or if they have taken their medications. Patients are theoretically at risk for prolonged effects if they receive benzodiazepines that are metabolized by the cytochrome P-450 system (see package insert for protease inhibitors). Midazolam and diazepam are metabolized by the P-450 system; lorazepam is glucuronidated.[25]

3. Elderly patients are at risk for becoming agitated, rather than sedated, by benzodiazepines. Flumazenil, a selective benzodiazepine antagonist, has been used to treat agitation during endoscopy resulting from benzodiazepine sedation;[18] however, finding alternative sedation would be a better proactive plan.

4. Oversedation with benzodiazepines can lead to airway obstruction from lax oropharyngeal tissues and poor control of the tongue in an unresponsive patient.

5. Oversedation by benzodiazepines, and sometimes even very small doses, can lead to hypotension.

Flumazenil, the specific antagonist, should be available whenever benzodiazepines are administered in order to enhance the safety of their use. It provides rapid reversal of oversedation.[25] Wille and colleagues[45] investigated routine rather than rescue use of flumazenil following upper endoscopy under midazolam. They were able to reduce recovery times in outpatients. However, when the cost of flumazenil was added to the bill, there were no cost savings for the shorter recovery period. At this time, there is no strong evidence suggesting a benefit to routine flumazenil use. There are, however, several drawbacks to its routine use. More than 10% of patients experience dizziness, nausea, and vomiting. Tremor, weakness, abnormal vision, dyspnea and hyperventilation, headache, and emotional disturbances can be a problem for 1–10% of patients.[25] Second, if a patient has received benzodiazepines routinely, use of flumazenil may precipitate withdrawal and seizures. Third, flumazenil is clinically effective for about 1 hour. If longer-lasting benzodiazepines are still present at this time, the patient will become resedated.

Analgesics

Pain control can be an important issue for endoscopy. Some procedures, such as esophageal dilation, are performed under general anesthesia for pain control. For other less painful procedures, such as colonoscopy, the addition of an analgesic agent to the sedation regimen is generally sufficient. Although several classes of analgesics are available, not all are appropriate for endoscopy. For example, ketorolac, a nonsteroidal antiinflamatory agent available for IV use, provides very good analgesia. It is not, however, appropriate for patients with suspected or known gastrointestinal bleeding or irritation, who represent a large portion of the endoscopy population. Narcotic analgesics are the most frequently used class of analgesics for endoscopy. They offer several advantages: (1) they provide excellent analgesia; (2) they are easily delivered IV, and their effects can be easily timed to coincide with procedural pain; (3) shorter-acting narcotics are available, decreasing recovery time; and (4) they only minimally alter hemodynamics in most situations. The most commonly used analgesics are meperidine or fentanyl. However, sufentanil and alfentanil have been used successfully.

Upper endoscopy is usually performed with only a sedative/anxiolytic such as a benzodiazepine. In a 1991 survey, 90% of endoscopists administered only an anxiolytic for most cases.[10] Only 13% of endoscopists added a narcotic analgesic. Studies have been divided on whether the addition of narcotics increases tolerance for the procedure.[12,40] Likewise, although it seems clear that topical oral anesthesia would increase patient comfort and tolerance, the results here are mixed as well.[7,27] Most endoscopists agree that sigmoidoscopy and colonoscopy are more painful for the patient than upper endoscopy. Use of narcotic analgesics is much more prevalent for these procedures when they are done under conscious sedation. There is no agreement on the best regimen and no agreement on whether an anxiolytic and/or an analgesic should be used. Some practitioners have used narcotics alone. DiPalma et al.[13] found that alfentanil alone did not differ from alfentanil and midazolam or meperidine and midazolam. Another study compared use of midazolam alone, pethidine (meperidine) alone, or midazolam plus pethidine. Patient acceptance and pain did not differ between groups.[17] Chokhavatia et al.[8] randomized patients to receive midazolam and one of the following four narcotics: meperidine, fentanyl, sufentanil, or alfentanil. Although sedation scores were higher with meperidine, so was patient comfort. While it is possible to provide good pain management with each of these narcotics, they have very different pharmacodynamic and pharmacokinetic profiles. This study suggests that it may be easier to do so with meperidine. Overall, the differing results of these studies suggest that there may be factors other than pharmacologic agents that result in patient comfort.

While narcotics provide outstanding analgesia, they have significant drawbacks that must be appreciated prior to their use. First and most problematic, they cause dose-dependent, centrally mediated respiratory depression that can lead to hypercapnia, narcosis, and apnea. Respiratory depression can occur with any narcotic agent. However, this is less likely to occur with less potent narcotics, such as meperidine, and narcotics that can be easily titrated, such as fentanyl. Most studies use one of these two agents for analgesia. An alternative strategy that has been considered is to use a shorter-acting narcotic agent such as alfentanil or remifentanyl; these agents produce clinical effects for only minutes after administration. However, they are also more likely to cause apnea, and have a smaller therapeutic window. All narcotics can produce other side effects such as nausea, vomiting, and pruritus.

Naloxone, the specific narcotic antagonist, should be available whenever narcotics are used. It is very effective in reversing respiratory depression, usually in very small doses. However, naloxone also can have adverse effects, such as hypertension, tachycardia, and onset of withdrawal.[25] Its routine administration to reverse acceptable levels of narcotic sedation is contraindicated.

Other Sedative Agents

Many other agents have been used for endoscopy. Benzodiazepines and narcotics usually provide very effective regimens with high patient satisfaction. However, both of these classes of agents produce tolerance. If a patient is taking oral narcotics or benzodiazepines at home, that class of medication will be less effective. Also, patients may be taking medications that have activated the P-450 system of the liver that metabolizes most of these agents. These medications commonly include antiseizure medications and alcohol.

Droperidol

When the usual regimens are not working or are not anticipated to work, the most common agent to add is droperidol. Droperidol is a butyrophenone that provides sedation and a state of dissociation or detachment. Unlike narcotics, droperidol does not depress respiratory drive. It can, however, cause prolonged sedation and dysphoria. In a study population in which 45% of patients had active alcohol use or withdrawal, the addition of droperidol to a benzodiazepine-narcotic regimen allowed a 98% procedure completion rate.[44] Several other studies show that the doses of benzodiazepines and narcotics can be decreased while patient tolerance remains good or improved;[4,36] however, patients remain sedated longer after the procedure. In the Rizzo study, patients actually had better tolerance for a relatively large-diameter endoscope for endoscopic ultrasound; however, the patients preferred sedation without droperidol. Others report the same dysphoria and extended sedation.[48]

Ketamine

Another useful sedative for difficult patients is ketamine. Ketamine is structurally related to phencyclidine and can produce very vivid and disturbing dreams. It also can easily cause increased sympathetic tone with hypertension, tachycardia, and increased oxygen demand.[25] Ketamine produces profound dose-dependent sedation and can be used as a general anesthetic. Its analgesia effects are also impressive, and are not cross-tolerant with narcotics. However, due to its effects on the cardiovascular system and the possible dysphoria, ketamine can be a difficult agent to use properly. If an agent such as ketamine is needed, a provider skilled in its use should be consulted.

Propofol

Propofol is a relatively new and very versatile intravenous anesthetic agent.[25] It is very useful for conscious sedation, and at higher doses it is an excellent general anesthetic. Patients find it to be very pleasant. Further, it is metabolized rapidly and has antiemetic properties. However, it does not have analgesic properties and therefore should be used in combination with narcotics for painful procedures.

The use of propofol for endoscopy by nonanesthesiologists is currently being debated in the literature. Propofol usually needs to be given as an infusion due to its rapid metabolism. It has a very narrow therapeutic range and can easily cause apnea requiring airway management whether given in bolus doses or as an infusion. The effects of propofol are synergistic with benzodiazepines and narcotics; therefore, respiratory depression and general anesthesia are even easier to produce unexpectedly. Propofol has been used successfully in colonoscopy. However, respiratory depression has been reported in some studies. Wehrmann et al.[43] prospectively compared the use of propofol with midazolam for endoscopic retrograde cholangiopancreatography (ERCP). Although patient cooperation was better in the propofol group, one patient required mask ventilation for 8 minutes of apnea. Although the use of propofol is increasing for endoscopy, many nonanesthesiologists as well as anesthesiologists feel that its use should be restricted to situations when airway experts are available.[5,20]

Nitrous Oxide

Nitrous oxide, an inhaled sedative and analgesic, has been administered as an alternative to IV sedation. Three studies carried out between 1994 and 1996 found it to be safe and effective. Recovery times were shorter, allowing earlier patient discharges.[29,32,39] Forbes et al.[16] compared the use of nitrous oxide to IV sedation/analgesia for colonoscopy. Patients were questioned about pain, tolerance, and satisfaction. Intravenous sedation with midazolam/meperidine was rated as significantly better in all categories than that with nitrous oxide. Further, endoscopists concurred that the nitrous oxide patients did not tolerate the procedure as well; however, they recovered more quickly. Overall, nitrous oxide should be considered an alternative sedative for colonoscopy, appropriate for carefuly selected patients. However, it does not appear to be as effective as IV sedation/analgesia. Nitrous oxide also carries the potential risk of inducing hypoxia, and should not necessarily be considered safer than IV sedation.

Patient-Controlled Sedation (PCS)

Several studies have recently reported on the feasibility of allowing patients to administer their own sedation, i.e., patient-controlled sedation (PCS). This is an adaptation of patient-controlled analgesia, a standard method for delivering IV pain medication to postoperative and chronic pain patients. A delivery system is programmed to allow the patient to push a button that initiates injection of a fixed amount of drug. The system limits how often an injection can occur and the dose of each injection, no matter how many times the button is pushed. When the patient is sedated and comfortable, he or she will not push the button, decreasing the likelihood of administering unneeded medication. This system is not foolproof and patients need to be carefully monitored; however, it has been a very effective delivery mode for postoperative pain.

Articles from the endoscopy literature suggest that patient-controlled delivery, or PCS, can work for procedural sedation as well. Stermer et al.[42] administered midazolam and meperidine to all patients prior to colonoscopy. During the procedure, additional meperidine was given either by an anesthesiologist or by PCS. Both methods were equally effective with respect to patient tolerance and safety. Roseveare et al.[38] compared use of propofol/alfentanil delivered by PCS with meperidine/diazepam delivered by standard administration for colonoscopy. The propofol/alfentanil group recovered more quickly, but reported more pain than the standard meperidine/diazepam group. Overall, although PCS has provided adequate sedation and analgesia, this method has not been shown to be superior to standard administration. At this point, cost savings by the PCS method have not been established.

Summary of Sedatives and Analgesics

Virtually all sedative and analgesic agents have been used during endoscopy. Clearly, some agents are easier to use than others and most have been shown to be consistently effective. Upper endoscopy (EGD) can be comfortably accomplished with only an anxiolytic. Lower endoscopy (colonoscopy) is generally considered more painful by patients. Studies show that patients undergoing lower endoscopy are consistently comfortable with a narcotic analgesic and an anxiolytic. However, practice and patient expectations are so variable that it is difficult to say that this sedation regimen is necessary for everyone, or even most patients. Endoscopists should seriously consider a sedation-as-needed strategy for select patients.

Keeping a simple, routine conscious sedation regimen is important for several reasons. Most sedatives and analgesics are synergistic; the margin of safety will decrease with multiple agents. Second, routine use of a few medications allows the endoscopist to become more familiar with the degree of expected sedation and what is unexpected from a particular medication. It is not as important to be versatile with several sedatives as it is to be safe and skilled with the administration of one. If a patient would be better off receiving a sedative with which the endoscopist is not familiar, a practitioner more familiar with its use should be consulted.

Practice Guidelines

The American Society of Anesthesiologists (ASA) has published practice guidelines for sedation and analgesia by nonanesthesiologists.[1] These guidelines are applicable to issues facing endoscopists and are discussed with endoscopists in mind. In addition, the American Society of Gastroenterology (ASGE) provides ongoing discussion of current practice guidelines at www.asge.org.

Patient Evaluation and Preparation

The literature suggests that a good preprocedural history and physical examination reduce the risk of adverse outcomes. Certain patient populations are at risk for complications during sedation. These include major organ dysfunction (particularly if poorly controlled), obesity, pregnancy, drug or alcohol abuse, and neurologic or psychiatric dysfunction rendering the patient uncooperative. Significant cardiopulmonary abnormalities, in particular, can put the patient at risk during sedation. If the patient has had general anesthesia or conscious sedation in the past, any adverse reactions or events should be explored. The endoscopist should be familiar with the patient's current medications and any herbal/nutritional supplements, drug allergies, tobacco and alcohol history, and any substance use. This history will help guide the use of, and help predict sensitivity to individual sedatives. Preprocedural laboratory evaluation depends on the health of the individual patient, and what effect the results might have on management of sedation. A physical examination should include heart, lungs, airway, and a gross evaluation of neurologic function. An airway evaluation should include adequacy of mouth opening (particularly visibility of the uvula), adequate thyromental distance, and neck size and flexibility. Limited mouth opening or a mouth occupied overwhelmingly by a large tongue, a short chin, and an inflexible neck are all predictors of problems with mask ventilation and tracheal intubation. Mild problems encountered by history or physical may simply suggest that a lighter sedation regimen should be considered. More serious problems may prompt the endoscopist to consult an anesthesiologist, and plan a different or better-monitored strategy for endoscopy.

One problem particular to upper endoscopy is the possibility of bleeding. If esophageal varices are present or suspected, the likelihood of bleeding is higher. During the procedure, massive bleeding could create an airway emergency requiring tracheal intubation. Endoscopists should consider whether these procedures should be done in a critical care setting, with patients intubated prior to the procedure. Airway management may require the presence of an intensivist or anesthesiologist. Triage with regard to location, monitoring strategy, and personnel is an important part of the preprocedural evaluation.

Patients undergoing sedation should undergo a discussion of the risks and benefits of sedation. They should also be given an opportunity to ask questions. The ASA suggests that patients not eat or drink for a period of time sufficient to empty the stomach. Generally, this period is considered to be 8 hours, although clear liquids empty in less time. The benefits of foregoing oral intake are not as clear for sedation as they are for general anesthesia. Under general anesthesia, airway reflexes are lost, and aspiration of stomach contents could easily occur. Presumably, airway reflexes remain intact during conscious sedation, but loss of consciousness with loss of reflexes may occur inadvertently during conscious sedation. Therefore, refraining from oral intake for 8 hours prior to the procedure is a good common-sense rule.

Intraprocedural Monitoring

Several specific areas of concern have been identified by the ASA practice guidelines for sedation: level of consciousness, pulmonary ventilation, oxygenation, and hemodynamics. These areas are reviewed briefly.

Level of Consciousness

A patient must be responsive to fulfill the definition of conscious sedation. If a patient becomes unresponsive, this is approaching general anesthesia. Airway reflexes can be lost; apnea, hypoxia, and hypercarbia may develop. The goal, instead, is to have a patient who is able to respond purposefully to verbal commands. If a patient can respond verbally, this provides a very good indication that the patient is breathing. If the patient cannot speak due to the particular procedure, following a command can help to assess the depth of sedation. If deep sedation with minimal responsiveness is reached, the patient should receive less or no more sedation at this point and be monitored carefully.

Ventilation

Sedation produces hypoventilation in several ways; central hypoventilation occurs and oropharyngeal obstruction of breathing decreases effective ventilation. The ASA Task Force suggests that this drug-induced respiratory depression is a primary cause of morbidity associated with sedation/analgesia given for procedures. Ventilation can be crudely monitored by following respiratory rate and effort, and by auscultating breath sounds. Certainly apnea can be distinguished by these methods. However, significant hypercarbia is harder to detect, since most patients will not have a concommitant decrease in O_2. Hypoxia actually develops later and would correlate with an extremely high CO_2. Nelson et al.[31] have studied the use of transcutaneous CO_2 monitoring and found that it prevented episodes of extreme hypercarbia (defined as > 40 mm Hg increase over baseline) in a significant number of patients. They further noted that these episodes were not reliably detected by clinical observation or by O_2 saturation monitoring. Unfortunately, outcome studies are not available to indicate how important CO_2 monitoring may be. However, individual practitioners may find it useful to use transcutaneous or nasal cannulae side-port CO_2 monitoring. In general, maintaining lighter sedation with an adequate respiratory rate and effort is the preferable solution for most patients. Although no standards have yet been set for use of CO_2 monitoring, this may be prudent in patients with underlying pulmonary disease.

Oxygenation

Oxygenation is typically measured by pulse oximetry. This method is easy, noninvasive, continuous, and accurate. Neither observation of respiratory rate and effort nor observation of patient skin tone is a substitute for monitoring oxygenation. Pulse oximetry is much more sensitive and detects problems much earlier.

Multiple studies have noted that oxygen desaturation occurs in a significant portion of patients who are undergoing upper and lower endoscopy without supplemental oxygen. Between 20% and 75% of sedated patients desaturate to less than 90% oxygen saturation (SaO_2), and often to less than 85%.[6,15,19] It seems likely that sedation is completely responsible for the desaturation. However, a portion of unsedated patients also experiences hypoxemia. Gombar et al.[19] randomized patients to receive diazepam or placebo premedication for upper endoscopy. Twenty percent of sedated and 10% of placebo patients experienced a SaO_2 less than 90% during endoscopy. Other studies have confirmed that a portion of patients will desaturate without sedation. In addition, some sedated patients will experience hypoxemia out of proportion to the level of sedation. Therefore, there may be factors other than sedation that contribute to hypoxemia.

Several recent patient series have identified risk factors that may predispose patients to desaturation during endoscopy. Alcain et al.[2] monitored 481 patients undergoing unsedated upper endoscopy. Six percent of these patients had a transient decrease in SaO_2 to less than 90%. Risk factors in these patients included ASA classification III or IV (i.e., significant coexisting disease that is not well controlled or is life-threatening), more than one attempt needed for esophageal probe intubation, emergency procedure, significant underlying respiratory disease, or a baseline SaO_2 less than 95%. Other studies have suggested additional independent risk factors: obesity, age greater than 65 years, anemia, and the level of experience of the endoscopist.[11,26,46,47]

Most of these studies concluded that the use of pulse oximetry is advisable, as does the ASA Task Force. Although improved outcome has not been demonstrated, transient hypoxia is extremely common and can usually be avoided or treated. Pulse oximetry should be considered standard of care, particularly in sicker populations.

The use of supplemental oxygen during endoscopy is highly advisable. Many studies from the gastrointestinal literature have shown that supplemental oxygen can prevent or reverse hypoxemia in endoscopy patients.[9,22] The ASA Task Force guidelines recommend that supplemental oxygen be immediately available whenever sedation/analgesia is administered. They recommend the use of oxygen whenever hypoxemia is anticipated or has developed. In light of the number of patients with hypoxemia even without sedation, supplemental oxygen should always be available when endoscopy is performed—with or without sedation. Further, many authors would argue that supplemental oxygen should always be used during endoscopy, whether or not its use is supported by outcome data.[5]

Patients with cardiac disease undergoing endoscopy pose a special challenge. These patients are more likely to experience ST segment changes during the procedure. It seems reasonable that these changes may be related to hypoxia. Jurell et al.[24] studied patients with cardiac disease undergoing endoscopy. They found less intraprocedural ST segment changes in patients who received supplemental oxygen. However, others have found no improvement in ST segment changes in this population related to oxygenation. Rosenberg et al.[37] found that tachycardia was a greater contributor to ST segment changes than hypoxia. In a separate study, they show that tachycardia occurs no less frequently in patients treated with supplemental oxygen.[23] Taken together, results of these studies suggest that tachycardia, as well as hypoxemia, should be controlled in patients with cardiac disease.

Hemodynamics

Vital signs, including blood pressure, heart rate, respiratory rate, and oxygen saturation should be monitored at regular intervals. Ideally, baseline data should be obtained before the procedure begins and before sedation is given. In the view of the ASA Task Force, sedation can blunt appropriate autonomic compensation for procedural stress or hypovolemia. Regular monitoring can detect hypotension early and avoid cardiovascular collapse. Further, patients with a cardiac history or advanced age should have electrocardiography (ECG) monitoring. Multiple studies have found that patients in these risk groups have a greater chance of experiencing the development or exacerbation of arrhythmias.[28,30]

Overall, the ASA recommends monitoring level of consciousness, ventilation, oxygenation, and hemodynamics. The Task Force recognizes the difficulty of providing this level of monitoring by one person alone. The endoscopist cannot perform the procedure and give adequate attention to monitoring. Instead, there should be another individual dedicated to monitoring. This individual also may assist the endoscopist to the extent that it does not interfere with patient monitoring. The patient needs to continue to be monitored post-procedure until the risk of cardiopulmonary depression has passed. Overall, this level of monitoring should improve patient comfort and satisfaction while reducing risk. The Task Force also strongly supports the view that emergency equipment for management of airway problems should be readily available. Pharmacologic emergency drugs, including flumazenil and naloxone, also should be available. In addition, the endoscopy should take place in a setting where further assistance, including an anesthesiologist or other ACLS provider, can be readily summoned.

Summary

Worldwide practices in the use of sedation for endoscopic procedures vary widely. Practice varies in the use of specific sedative agents, and even whether sedation is used at all. It appears, however, that endoscopic procedures are generally better tolerated with sedation. This is particularly true in countries such as the United States where the expectation of receiving sedation is almost universal. However, sedation is not always a necessity, and select patients may feel differently with education and the option of "sedation only as needed." The task of the endoscopist is to provide good patient education and to provide appropriate choices. When sedation is indicated, the task of the endoscopist is to provide comfort by administering safe sedation. Sedated or unsedated, safe endoscopy begins with good preprocedural screening and selection of appropriate patient populations. Safe practice continues with an endoscopist who is knowledgeable about and comfortable with sedatives and sedation practices. Safe practice also includes adequate monitoring and emergency equipment and personnel availability. For patients with extensive coexisting disease or other problems of an unusual nature, safe practice dictates consulting and using a sedation specialist such as an anesthesiologist or intensivist. Endoscopy will probably continue to become more tolerable and even comfortable without sedation, as the use of small-caliber endoscopes increases. Sedation may become a much more selective practice in the future.

References

1. American Society of Anesthesiologists: Practice guidelines for sedation and analgesia by non-anesthesiologists. A report by the American Society of Anesthesiologists Task Force on Sedation and Analgesia by Non-Anesthesiologists. Anesthesiology 84:459–471, 1996.

2. Alcain G, Guillen P, Escolar A, et al: Predictive factors of oxygen desaturation during upper gastrointestinal endoscopy in nonsedated patients. Gastrointest Endosc 48:143–147, 1998.

3. Arrowsmith JB, Gerstman BB, Fleischer DE, Benjamin SB: Results from the American Society for Gastrointestinal Endoscopy/U.S. Food and Drug Administration collaborative study on complication rates and drug use during gastrointestinal endoscopy. Gastrointest Endosc 37:421–427, 1991.

4. Barthel JS, Marshall JB, King PD, et al: The effect of droperidol on objective markers of patient cooperation and vital signs during esophagogastroduodenoscopy: A randomized, double-blind, placebo-controlled, prospective investigation [published erratum appears in Gastrointest Endosc 42:385, 1995]. Gastrointest Endosc 42:45–50, 1995.

5. Bell GD, Charlton JE: Colonoscopy: Is sedation necessary and is there any role for intravenous propofol? [editorial comment]. Endoscopy 32:264–267, 2000.

6. Bowton DL, Scuderi PE, Harris L, Haponik EF: Pulse oximetry monitoring outside the intensive care unit: Progress or problem? Ann Intern Med 115:450–454, 1991.

7. Cantor DS, Baldridge ET: Premedication with meperidine and diazepam for upper gastrointestinal endoscopy precludes the need for topical anesthesia. Gastrointest Endosc 32:339–341, 1986.

8. Chokhavatia S, Nguyen L, Williams R, et al: Sedation and analgesia for gastrointestinal endoscopy. Am J Gastroenterol 88:393–396, 1993.

9. Crantock L, Cowen AE, Ward M, Roberts RK: Supplemental low flow oxygen prevents hypoxia during endoscopic cholangiopancreatography. Gastrointest Endosc 38:418–420, 1992.

10. Daneshmend TK, Bell GD, Logan RF: Sedation for upper gastrointestinal endoscopy: Results of a nationwide survey. Gut 32:12–15, 1991.

11. Dhariwal A, Plevris JN, Lo NT, et al: Age, anemia, and obesity-associated oxygen desaturation during upper gastrointestinal endoscopy. Gastrointest Endosc 38:684–688, 1992.

12. Diab FH, King PD, Barthel JS, Marshall JB: Efficacy and safety of combined meperidine and midazolam for EGD sedation compared with midazolam alone. Am J Gastroenterol 91:1120–1125, 1996.

13. DiPalma JA, Herrera JL, Weis FR, et al: Alfentanil for conscious sedation during colonoscopy. South Med J 88:630–634, 1995.

14. Eckardt VF, Kanzier G, Willems D, et al: Colonoscopy without premedication versus barium enema: A comparison of patient discomfort. Gastrointest Endosc 44:177–180, 1996.

15. Fassoulaki A, Mihas A: Changes in arterial blood gases associated with gastrointestinal endoscopies. Acta Anaesthesiol Belg 38:127–131, 1987.

16. Forbes GM, Collins BJ: Nitrous oxide for colonoscopy: A randomized controlled study. Gastrointest Endosc 51:271–277, 2000.

17. Froehlich F, Thorens J, Schwizer W, et al: Sedation and analgesia for colonoscopy: Patient tolerance, pain, and cardiorespiratory parameters. Gastrointest Endosc 45:1–9, 1997.

18. Fulton SA, Mullen KD: Completion of upper endoscopic procedures despite paradoxical reaction to midazolam: A role for flumazenil? Am J Gastroenterol 95:809–811, 2000.

19. Gombar KK, Dhall JC, Suri RP, et al: Effect of diazepam sedation on arterial oxygen saturation during esophagogastroduodenoscopy: A placebo-controlled study. Indian J Gastroenterol 15:40–42, 1996.

20. Graber RG: Propofol in the endoscopy suite: An anesthesiologist's perspective [editorial comment]. Gastrointest Endosc 49:803–806, 1999.

21. Greff M: Colorectal cancer screening in France: Guidelines and professional reality [editorial]. Endoscopy 31:471, 1999.

22. Gross JB, Long WB: Nasal oxygen alleviates hypoxemia in colonoscopy patients sedated with midazolam and meperidine. Gastrointest Endosc 36:26–29, 1990.

23. Holm C, Christensen M, Schulze S, Rosenberg J: Effect of oxygen on tachycardia and arterial oxygen saturation during colonoscopy. Eur J Surg 165:755–758, 1999.

24. Jurell KR, O'Connor KW, Slack J, et al: Effect of supplemental oxygen on cardiopulmonary changes during gastrointestinal endoscopy. Gastrointest Endosc 40:665–670, 1994.

25. Lacy C, Armstrong L, Ingrim N, Lance L: Drug Information Handbook, 5th ed. Hudson, Lexi-Comp Inc., 1997.

26. Lavies NG, Creasy T, Harris K, Hanning CD: Arterial oxygen saturation during upper gastrointestinal endoscopy: Influence of sedation and operator experience. Am J Gastroenterol 83:618–622, 1988.

27. Leitch DG, Wicks J, el Beshir OA, et al: Topical anesthesia with 50 mg of lidocaine spray facilitates upper gastrointestinal endoscopy. Gastrointest Endosc 39:384–387, 1993.

28. Lieberman DA, Wuerker CK, Katon RM: Cardiopulmonary risk of esophagogastroduodenoscopy: Role of endoscope diameter and systemic sedation. Gastroenterology 88:468–472, 1985.

29. Lindblom A, Jansson O, Jeppsson B, et al: Nitrous oxide for colonoscopy discomfort: A randomized double-blind study. Endoscopy 26:283–286, 1994.

30. McAlpine JK, Martin BJ, Devine BL: Cardiac arrhythmias associated with upper gastrointestinal endoscopy in elderly subjects. Scott Med J 35:102–104, 1990.

31. Nelson DB, Freeman ML, Silvis SE, et al: A randomized, controlled trial of transcutaneous carbon dioxide monitoring during ERCP. Gastrointest Endosc 51:288–295, 2000.

32. Notini-Gudmarsson AK, Dolk A, Jakobsson J, Johansson C: Nitrous oxide: A valuable alternative for pain relief and sedation during routine colonoscopy. Endoscopy 28:283–287, 1996.

33. Quine MA, Bell GD, McCloy RF, et al: Prospective audit of upper gastrointestinal endoscopy in two regions of England: Safety, staffing, and sedation methods. Gut 36:462–467, 1995.

34. Rex DK, Imperiale TF, Portish V: Patients willing to try colonoscopy without sedation: Associated clinical factors and results of a randomized controlled trial. Gastrointest Endosc 49:554–559, 1999.

35. Ristikankare M, Hartikainen J, Heikkinen M, et al: Is routinely given conscious sedation of benefit during colonoscopy? Gastrointest Endosc 49:566–572, 1999.

36. Rizzo J, Bernstein D, Gress F: A randomized double-blind placebo-controlled trial evaluating the cost-effectiveness of droperidol as a sedative premedication for EUS. Gastrointest Endosc 50:178–182, 1999.

37. Rosenberg J, Stausholm K, Andersen IB, et al: No effect of oxygen therapy on myocardial ischaemia during gastroscopy. Scand J Gastroenterol 31:200–205, 1996.

38. Roseveare C, Seavell C, Patel P, et al: Patient-controlled sedation and analgesia, using propofol and alfentanil, during colonoscopy: A prospective randomized controlled trial. Endoscopy 30:768–773, 1998.

39. Saunders BP, Fukumoto M, Halligan S, et al: Patient-administered nitrous oxide/oxygen inhalation provides effective sedation and analgesia for colonoscopy. Gastrointest Endosc 40:418–421, 1994.

40. Schwartz SE, Fazio TL: Pre-endoscopic medication: A randomized double-blind trial of atropine and meperidine as a supplement to diazepam. Scand J Gastroenterol 14:747–751, 1979.

41. Sorbi D, Gostout CJ, Henry J, Lindor KD: Unsedated small-caliber esophagogastroduodenoscopy (EGD) versus conventional EGD: A comparative study. Gastroenterology 117:1301–1307, 1999.

42. Stermer E, Gaitini L, Yudashkin M, et al: Patient-controlled analgesia for conscious sedation during colonoscopy: A randomized controlled study. Gastrointest Endosc 51:278–281, 2000.

43. Wehrmann T, Kokabpick S, Lembcke B, et al: Efficacy and safety of intravenous propofol sedation during routine ERCP: A prospective, controlled study. Gastrointest Endosc 49:677–683, 1999.

44. Wilcox CM, Forsmark CE, Cello JP: Utility of droperidol for conscious sedation in gastrointestinal endoscopic procedures. Gastrointest Endosc 36:112–115, 1990.

45. Wille RT, Chaffee BW, Ryan ML, et al: Pharmacoeconomic evaluation of flumazenil for routine outpatient EGD. Gastrointest Endosc 51:282–287, 2000.

46. Woods SD, Chung SC, Leung JW, et al: Hypoxia and tachycardia during endoscopic retrograde cholangiopancreatography: Detection by pulse oximetry. Gastrointest Endosc 35:523–525, 1989.

47. Yano H, Iishi H, Tatsuta M, et al: Oxygen desaturation during sedation for colonoscopy in elderly patients. Hepatogastroenterology 45:2138–2141, 1998.

48. Zuccaro G Jr: Sedation and sedationless endoscopy. Gastrointest Endosc Clin North Am 10:1–20, 2000.

10

Conscious Sedation for Assisted Reproductive Technologies

Lynn M. Westphal, M.D.
Stephen B. Mooney, M.D.

Assisted reproductive technology refers to all fertility treatments that involve direct retrieval of oocytes from the ovaries. In vitro fertilization (IVF) involves ovarian stimulation to induce multiple follicle growth, oocyte extraction, laboratory fertilization of oocytes, and transfer of embryos into the uterus. Gamete intrafallopian transfer (GIFT) refers to oocyte retrieval followed immediately by the placement of oocytes and sperm into the fallopian tube. Zygote intrafallopian transfer (ZIFT) and tubal embryo transfer (TET) involve the placement of fertilized oocytes/embryos into the fallopian tube. GIFT, ZIFT, and TET are usually done by laparoscopy. Since GIFT, ZIFT, and TET are more invasive and prospective comparisons show no benefit in pregnancy rate,[2,35] these procedures are rarely done. The most recent statistics show that only about 5% of procedures in the U.S. involve GIFT or ZIFT.[8]

Coincident with efforts to increase pregnancy rates with IVF have been the strides made to simplify and optimize the various steps of the overall IVF procedure. Since 1978, when the first "test tube" baby was born through the IVF technique,[33] several refinements in IVF techniques have occurred. One of the improvements has been the simplification of the oocyte extraction process. Oocyte aspiration was originally performed by direct visualization of the ovary at laparoscopy.[22] Later, transvesical oocyte retrieval was accomplished with abdominal ultrasound guidance.[14] During the late 1980s, transvaginal oocyte aspiration for IVF became routine in many centers.[12,18] In addition to being a procedure of shorter duration, transvaginal oocyte retrieval has been associated with higher fertilization rates than laparoscopic oocyte retrieval.[36] Moreover, the relative ease of transvaginal oocyte retrieval has encouraged its performance outside the operating room setting. These changes in IVF have called for adjustments in anesthetic technique in order to improve the patient's experience and diminish the procedure's cost. These matters are especially important with the realization that some patients may undergo oocyte retrieval several times before they conceive.

Although generally lasting only 20–30 minutes, transvaginal oocyte retrieval involves passing a needle through the vaginal wall in order to puncture and aspirate the ovarian follicles. Typically, the discomfort is most intense upon initial entry of the ovary, and there is usually little additional pain with intraovarian maneuvers of the needle. Without adequate anesthesia or analgesia, the patient can be very uncomfortable. Obviously, if the patient is moving, the procedure is also much more difficult to complete safely. Thus, despite modifications in the oocyte extraction process, some form of analgesia or anesthesia remains the standard of care.

A variety of anesthetic techniques have been used to make transvaginal oocyte retrieval safe and efficient. Although general, regional, and local anesthetic methods have all been successfully employed during oocyte aspiration, conscious sedation has emerged as the most widely used anesthetic technique for this procedure. Ditkoff et al.[12] conducted a survey of programs of the Society of Assisted Reproductive Technology (SART) regarding the use of anesthesia for oocyte retrieval. All respondents reported the use of some type of intravenous (IV) sedation, with 95% of programs preferring the use of conscious sedation. Several SART programs did not use specific anesthesia personnel to provide the conscious sedation. For this reason, these centers primarily used midazolam and meperidine during oocyte retrievals, whereas those using anesthesia staff commonly administered propofol and/or fentanyl for conscious sedation.

The objective of this chapter is to review the principles and practice of anesthesia care of the infertile patient and present the practitioner with recommendations for the rational use of conscious sedation in patients undergoing oocyte retrieval procedures for IVF. Our recommendations originate from data published on clinical reproductive medicine and general pharmacology as well as personal experiences with administration of conscious sedation for IVF.

Types of Anesthesia for Transvaginal Follicle Aspiration

Oocyte retrievals are relatively short procedures that are performed on an outpatient basis and are often done outside a standard operating room. The optimal anesthetic technique should result in few side effects, a short recovery time, and be nontoxic to the oocytes that are being recovered. The types of anesthesia used for transvaginal oocyte retrieval have included general, spinal, and epidural anesthesia, conscious sedation, local injection, or no anesthesia at all. Accordingly, each anesthetic method has its inherent advantages and disadvantages.

General Anesthesia

General anesthesia usually results in a longer recovery time, with a significant risk of nausea or other side effects. In addition to requiring an anesthesiologist for administration, general anesthesia requires access to complex and costly monitoring equipment. It is well known that general anesthetics rapidly traverse into the follicular fluid during their administration for oocyte retrieval.[32,37] Many authors have postulated that this may be responsible for detrimental effects seen on cleavage rates of embryos[13,19,21,25] and pregnancy rates.[15,16] Fishel et al. compared enflurane and halothane and found that halothane significantly reduced the incidence of implantation.[15] Boyer et al. noted that cleavage rates declined in oocytes that were obtained later during general anesthesia.[4] They questioned whether the accumulation of general anesthetic agents in follicular fluid may have caused this phenomenon. Furthermore, a greater transient rise in prolactin levels has been reported with general anesthesia as compared to the rise associated with IV sedation.[30] Since lowering the prolactin level with bromocriptine has been shown to enhance cleavage rates, it follows that an increased prolactin level could affect the IVF outcome.[31]

Regional Anesthesia

The use of epidural anesthesia can avoid many of the side effects of general anesthesia[20] and shortens recovery time.[23] For IVF, epidural anesthesia may be more advantageous than general anesthesia because it results in lower levels of anesthetic agents in the follicular fluid. On the other hand, when epidural anesthesia was compared with IV sedation and mask ventilation, Botta et al.[5] found no difference in the IVF pregnancy rates. Of note, the costs related to the expertise of an anesthesiologist plus the necessary specialized equipment may deter some programs from using epidural anesthesia.

Since a local anesthetic agent can anesthetize only the vaginal mucosa and not the ovary itself, the application of local anesthesia is usually not adequate for pain relief.[3] Furthermore, patients are often anxious and may be uncomfortable being in lithotomy position for 20–30 minutes. Bailey-Pridham et al.[1] demonstrated the presence of pharmacologic levels of lidocaine in human serum and follicular fluid of eight patients, but four conceived, so it did not appear to be significant. Another study looked at fertilization and cleavage rates and found no difference between patients that received a paracervical block with lidocaine and those who did not.[39] A recent study looked at the efficacy of paracervical block in combination with intravenous sedation and noted a decrease in the abdominal pain that patients reported during the procedure.[27] However, an earlier study[11] showed that in patients receiving intravenous sedation, there was no difference between paracervical block and no injection in terms of global pain evaluation.

Spinal anesthesia has been used routinely at some institutions. Viscomi et al.[38] report a shorter recovery time for spinal anesthesia compared to conscious sedation. However, their study was not randomized, and data are from procedures in

1993–1994, when operative times were longer. They report two admissions for uncontrolled nausea and vomiting (in the conscious sedation group) and one post–spinal anesthesia headache. Martin and colleagues[24] looked at the possibility of decreasing recovery times after spinal anesthesia. They showed that when fentanyl was added to 1.5% lidocaine for spinal anesthesia, patients were more comfortable during the procedure and required less narcotics postoperatively.

Conscious Sedation

Conscious sedation is well tolerated by patients, does not require specialized equipment, and is associated with a low incidence of complications. The overall rate of complications has been reported at 0.16% for IVF; most of the complications recorded were intra-abdominal bleeding and, thus, not seemingly related to the anesthesia method itself.[28] With conscious sedation, the perception of pain during transvaginal oocyte retrieval was similar to that experienced with cervical dilatation or hysterosalpingography.[17] The study by Ditkoff et al.[12] has documented a widespread acceptance of conscious sedation for oocyte retrieval procedures. The frequency of this practice among SART IVF programs points out that programs find it easy to use, economical, and effective.

Like general anesthesia, conscious sedation shares the risk that follicular fluid may be contaminated by anesthetic agents during oocyte retrieval. Studies addressing this concern have shown no negative effect with respect to the agents used for conscious sedation. In early work, Bruce et al.[6] studied the effect of fentanyl on sea urchin eggs; no detrimental effects on fertilization and development were discovered. Likewise, Swanson and Leavitt,[34] in their study using midazolam, could not find any effect on mouse embryos. Furthermore, after IV administration midazolam could not be found in the follicular fluid of women.[9] Although propofol accumulates in follicular fluid,[29] no difference in fertilization, embryo cleavage, or implantation rates were seen when compared to paracervical block.[10] Propofol and low-dose fentanyl have been compared to midazolam and remifentanil and no differences in safety and efficacy were seen.[7] The need for face mask ventilation was seen more frequently in those receiving fentanyl/propofol, but all patients would accept the same treatment in a future cycle. Patients receiving remifentanil had a higher incidence of intraoperative recall and 13% said they would not accept the same anesthetic regimen.

Conscious sedation does not seem to cause the increase in prolactin previously associated with general anesthesia.[30] Interestingly, the possibility exists that agents used in combination may have drawbacks, thus potentially affecting the outcome of IVF. For instance, the combination of droperidol and fentanyl reportedly increased prolactin levels and lead to decreased progesterone levels in the luteal phase of patients undergoing transvaginal follicle aspiration for IVF.[26]

The "perfect" anesthetic method would have the following attributes: (1) it would be highly effective and very safe; (2) it would be easy for practitioners to administer, monitor, and reverse; (3) it would be short-acting and elicit the fewest side effects yet provide adequate sedation and analgesia. Since many anesthetic agents have been detected in follicular fluid within minutes after administration,[32] the "perfect" anesthetic to be used in IVF would be nontoxic to oocytes or embryos alike; thus, the overall goal of IVF, to establish a viable pregnancy, would not be undermined. With the knowledge that many patients have to pay for IVF services out-of-pocket, economic factors also must be considered when selecting the ideal type of anesthesia.

Despite the potential drawbacks and controversies noted above, conscious sedation appears to be the most ideal type of anesthesia for the relief of pain and discomfort during oocyte recovery. In our institution, this is usually performed with the administration of propofol and fentanyl.

Conclusion

Anesthesia that is safe, effective, short-acting, and economical has helped to encourage relatively recent changes in oocyte collection techniques. Conscious sedation has proven to be the anesthetic method nearest to ideal for most patients undergoing oocyte retrieval for IVF. Several authors have confirmed its efficacy and safety for oocyte harvest. Since the relatively short-acting agents used for conscious sedation provide rapidly reversible sedation and analgesia, post-retrieval recovery from conscious sedation tends to be short without lingering side effects; thus, patients return to routine activities more quickly. Compared to the costs of administering general or epidural anesthesia, conscious sedation costs are quite reasonable. For these reasons, the routine use of conscious sedation has been a catalyst in moving oocyte retrieval procedures out of the hospital setting.

Despite the apparent ideal nature of conscious sedation for IVF, some words of caution seem worthwhile regarding the use of this type of anesthesia. Some conscious sedation agents are known to rapidly traverse into the follicular fluid during oocyte retrieval. Although toxicity information from studies in humans has been generally reassuring, a few animal studies have provided contradictory results. While SART maintains statistical data on IVF success rates, including oocyte retrieval data, fertilization results, pregnancy rates, and birth rates, it does not collect information regarding complications of anesthesia during IVF procedures. Thus the currently available information regarding the safety and efficacy of conscious sedation relies upon data published by independent authors. Over time, reproductive endocrinologists and anesthesiologists alike have learned to successfully adapt the experiences of physicians in other specialties to conscious sedation for IVF procedures. However, due to the possibility of side effects and complications with any type of anesthesia used, physicians and other practitioners providing conscious sedation are required to be knowledgeable about the properties of the anesthetic agents they are administering. Therefore, conscious sedation is only feasible if adequately trained personnel is available to respond quickly and accurately in the event that complications occur.

References

1. Bailey-Pridham D, Reshef E, Durry K, et al: Follicular fluid lidocaine levels during oocyte retrieval. Fertil Steril 53:1710–1713, 1990.

2. Balmaseda JP, Alam V, Roszjteine D, et al: Embryo implantation rates in oocyte donation: A prospective comparison of tubal versus uterine transfers. Fertil Steril 57:365, 1992.

3. Ben-Shlomo I, Amodai I, Levran D, et al: Midazolam-fentanyl sedation in conjunction with local anesthesia during oocyte retrieval for in vitro fertilization. J Assist Reprod Genet 9:83–85, 1992.

4. Boyer SP, Lavy G, Russel JB, DeCherney AH: A paired analysis of in vitro fertilization and cleavage rates of first- versus last-recovered preovulatory human oocytes exposed to varying intervals of 100% CO_2 pneumoperitoneum and general anesthesia. Fertil Steril 48:969–974, 1987.

5. Botta G, D'Angelo A, D'Ari G, et al: Epidural anesthesia in an in vitro fertilization and embryo transfer program. J Assist Reprod Genet 12:187–190, 1995.

6. Bruce DL, Hinkley R, Norman PF: Fentanyl does not inhibit fertilization or early development of sea urchin eggs. Anesth Analg 64:498–500, 1985.

7. Casati A, Valentini G, Zangrillo A, et al: Anaesthesia for ultrasound guided oocyte retrieval: Midazolam/remifentanil versus propofol/fentanyl regimens. Eur J Anaesth 16:773–778, 1999.

8. Centers for Disease Control and Prevention: 1997 Assisted Reproductive Technology Success Rates. Atlanta, GA, Centers for Disease Control and Prevention, 1999.

9. Chopineau J, Bazin JE, Terrisse MP, et al: Assay for midazolam in liquor folliculi during in vitro fertilization under anesthesia. Clin Pharm 12:770–773, 1993.

10. Christiaens F, Moerman I, Janssenswillen C, et al: Accumulation of propofol in follicular fluid during transvaginal oocyte retrieval. Br J Anaesth 76:86–87, 1996.

11. Corson SL, Batzer FR, Gocial B, et al: Is paracervical block anesthesia for oocyte retrieval effective? Fertil Steril 62:133–136, 1994.

12. Ditkoff EC, Plumb J, Selick A, Sauer MV: Anesthesia practices in the United States common to in vitro fertilization (IVF) centers. J Assist Reprod Genet 14:145–147, 1997.

13. Endler GC, Stout M, Magyar DM, et al: Follicular fluid concentration of thiopental and thiamylal during laparoscopy for oocyte retrieval. Fertil Steril 48:828–833, 1987.

14. Feichtinger W: Current technique of oocyte retrieval. Curr Opin Obstet Gynecol 4:697–701, 1992.

15. Fishel S, Webster J, Faratian B, Jackson J: General anesthesia for intrauterine placement of human conceptuses after in vitro fertilization. J In Vitro Fert Embryo Transf 4:260–264, 1987.

16. Gonen O, Shulman A, Ghetler Y, et al: The impact of different types of anesthesia on in vitro fertilization: Embryo transfer treatment outcome. J Assist Reprod Genet 12:678–682, 1995.

17. Gohar J, Lunenfeld E, Potashik G, Glezerman M: The use of sedation only during oocyte retrieval for in vitro fertilization: Patients' pain self-assessments versus doctors' evaluations. J Assist Reprod Genet 10:476–478, 1993.

18. Hammarberg K, Enk L, Wilson L, Wikland M: Oocyte retrieval under guidance of a vaginal transducer: Evaluation of patients' acceptance. Hum Reprod 2:487–490, 1987.

19. Hayes MF, Sacco AG, Savoy-Moore RT, et al: Effect of general anesthesia on fertilization and cleavage of human oocytes in vitro. Fertil Steril 48:975–981, 1987.

20. Kogosowki A, Lessing JB, Amit A, et al: Epidural block: A preferred method of anesthesia for ultrasonically guided oocyte retrieval. Fertil Steril 47:166–168, 1987.

21. Lefebvre G, Vauthier D, Seebacher J, et al: In vitro fertilization: A comparative study of cleavage rates under epidural and general anesthesia: Interest for gamete intrafallopian transfer. J In Vitro Fert Embryo Transf 5:305–306, 1988.

22. Lewin A, Laufer N, Rabinowitz R, et al: Ultrasonically guided oocyte collection under local anesthesia: The first choice method for in vitro fertilization: A comparative study with laparoscopy. Fertil Steril 46:257–261, 1986.

23. Manica VS, Bader AM, Fragneto R, et al: Anesthesia for in vitro fertilization: A comparison of 1.5% and 5% spinal lidocaine for ultrasonically guided oocyte retrieval. Anesth Analg 77:453–456, 1993.

24. Martin R, Tsen LC, Tzeng G, et al: Anesthesia for in vitro fertilization: The addition of fentanyl to 1.5% lidocaine. Anesth Analg 88:523–526, 1999.

25. Matt DW, Steingold KA, Dastvan CM, et al: Effects of sera from patients given various anesthetics on preimplantation mouse embryo development in vitro. J In Vitro Fert Embryo Transf 8:191–197, 1991.

26. Naito Y, Tamai S, Fukata J, et al: Comparison of endocrinologic stress response associated with transvaginal ultrasound-guided oocyte pick-up under halothane anaesthesia and neuroleptanaesthesia. Can J Anaesth 36:633–636, 1989.

27. Ng EH, Tang OS, Chui DK, Ho PC: A prospective, randomized, double-blind and placebo-controlled study to assess the efficacy of paracervical block in the pain relief during egg collection in IVF. Hum Reprod 14:2783–2787, 1999.

28. Oskowitz SP, Berger MJ, Mullen L, et al: Safety of a freestanding surgical unit for the assisted reproductive technologies. Fertil Steril 63:874–879, 1995.

29. Palot M, Harika C, Pigeon F, et al: Propofol in general anesthesia for IVF (by vaginal and transurethral route): Follicular fluid concentration and cleavage rate. Anesthesiology 69:573, 1988.

30. Robinson JN, Forman RG, Lockwood GM, et al: A comparison of the transient hyperprolactineamic stress response obtained using two different methods of analgesia for ultrasound-guided transvaginal oocyte retrieval. Hum Reprod 6:1291–1293, 1991.

31. Sopelak VM, Whitworth NS, Norman PF, Cowan BD: Bromocriptine inhibition of anesthesia-induced hyperprolactinemia: Effects on serum and follicular fluid hormones, oocyte fertilization, and embryo cleavage rates during in vitro fertilization. Fertil Steril 52:627–632, 1989.

32. Soussis I, Boyd O, Paraschos T, et al: Follicular fluid levels of midazolam, fentanyl, and alfentanil during transvaginal oocyte retrieval. Fertil Steril 64:1003–1007, 1995.

33. Steptoe PC, Edwards RG: Birth after the reimplantation of a human embryo (letter). Lancet 2:366, 1978.

34. Swanson RJ, Leavitt MG: Fertilization and mouse embryo development in the presence of midazolam. Anesth Analg 75:549–554, 1992.

35. Tanbo T, Dale PO, Aabynolm T: Assisted fertilization in infertility women with patent fallopian tubes: A comparison of in vitro fertilizations gamete intrafallopian transfer and tubal embryo stage transfer. Hum Reprod 5:266–270, 1990.

36. Tanbo T, Henriksen T, Magnus O, Abyholm T: Oocyte retrieval in an IVF program: A comparison of laparoscopic and transvaginal ultrasound-guided follicular puncture. Acta Obst Gynacol Scand 67:243–246, 1988.
37. Trapp M, Baukloh V, Bohnet HG, Heeschen W: Pollutants in human follicular fluid. Fertil Steril 42:146–148, 1984.
38. Viscomi CM, Hill K, Sites C: Spinal anesthesia versus intravenous sedation for transvaginal oocyte retrieval reproductive outcome, side effects and recovery profiles. Int J Obstet Anaesth 6:49–51, 1997.
39. Wikland M, Evers H, Jakobsson AH, et al: The concentration of lidocaine in follicular fluid when used for paracervical block in a human IVF-ET programme. Hum Reprod 5:920–923, 1990.

11

Nursing Issues in Conscious Sedation

Miranda Kramer, MS, RN, NP, CCRN

As science and technology advance, so does nursing practice. Hospitalized patients are of a higher acuity than ever before and more high-tech procedures are performed on an outpatient basis. The nursing management of patients receiving conscious sedation applies to a multitude of health care environments and nurse roles. A variety of nursing positions now includes a component related to conscious sedation. Conscious sedation may be called for in the endoscopy suite, outpatient clinic, cardiac catheterization lab, emergency room, intensive care unit, or radiology department. Yet, one common factor in all these settings is that before, during, and after the procedure the patients will be cared for by a registered nurse.

By definition, "intravenous conscious sedation is produced by the administration of pharmacologic agents. A patient under conscious sedation has a depressed level of consciousness, but retains the ability to independently and continuously maintain a patent airway and respond appropriately to physical stimulation and/or verbal command".[1] This must be differentiated from "deep sedation," a medically controlled condition in which the patient has a depressed state of consciousness and is not arousable to command. A partial or complete loss of protective reflexes accompanies deep sedation, which is outside the realm of conscious sedation. Conscious sedation provides sedation and analgesia, which allows patients to tolerate unpleasant procedures while maintaining adequate cardiopulmonary function and response to stimuli.[3]

The goals of administration of conscious sedation include the following: alteration of mood, maintenance of consciousness, enhanced cooperation, elevation of the pain threshold, minimal variation of vital signs, some degree of amnesia and a rapid, safe return to activities of daily living.[3]

Before the Procedure

Once the client reaches the health care setting, the nurse–patient relationship begins. The nurse roles encompassed do not only include providing physiologic stability and safety but also advocacy and education. The nurse should evaluate the patient's anxiety level and prepare the patient for the events involved in the procedure. A patient who is overtly anxious, has special developmental needs, or is unable to provide informed consent is not a candidate for conscious sedation. The physician should be notified at once if these circumstances exist. Alternate forms of sedation and analgesia or rescheduling a procedure may be warranted. The patient's perceptions about the procedure and receiving conscious sedation should be clarified before any therapy is started. Providing clear instruction on what the patient will encounter allays anxieties and may decrease the amount of sedating medication needed to perform the procedure.[6] A calm, supportive nurse is immensely reassuring to the patient undergoing conscious sedation.

Physiologic conditions may preclude the use of conscious sedation outside the operating room. These conditions may include, but are not limited to, patients with difficult airway situations, morbid obesity, cardiopulmonary disease, unstable cardiac arrhythmias, or a history of untoward reaction to sedatives or analgesics. Renal or hepatic impairment may alter drug metabolism and clearance, which may make another form of sedation more appropriate.

Assessment

The nurse then performs the physical exam and reviews the patient's history. The nursing history includes the patient's allergies, current medication, previous response to analgesics and sedatives, tobacco and substance abuse history,

TABLE 1. The ASA Physical Status Classification System[2]

Class	Definition
1	Normal, healthy patient
2	Patient with mild systemic disease
3	Patient with severe systemic disease
4	Patient with severe systemic disease that is a constant threat to life
5	Moribund patient who is not expected to survive without the operation
6	Declared brain-dead patient whose organs are being removed for donor purposes
E	The letter "E" should follow in cases in which the patient was not scheduled for surgery, i.e., procedures done on an emergency basis

and past medical history. The nurse should also confirm the chief complaint and planned procedure with the patient. Accessory data obtained should include the appropriate laboratory data (blood count, baseline ECG). The patient's height, weight, and baseline vital signs will assist in guiding dosage of medications prescribed. The amount of time the patient has been NPO must be confirmed as well to prevent aspiration.

Many institutions have adopted the American Society of Anesthesiologists (ASA) classification of physical status in assessing a patient's appropriateness for conscious sedation (Table 1).

Patients with ASA classification 1 or 2 are candidates for conscious sedation. Those with classification 3 or 4 are referred to an anesthesiologist for further evaluation due to physical conditions that place them at greater risk for complications. Patients with classification 5 and 6 are also unsuitable candidates for conscious sedation because it is not clinically indicated. The Mallampati scale should also be used to rate a patient's airway. The Mallampati classification system is useful in predicting patients with difficult airway situations.[5]

Patient Preparation

Once the patient has given informed consent and is ready for the procedure, the nurse arranges to begin the procedure. This starts with placing the patient on cardiac, blood pressure, and pulse oximetry monitoring. Pulse oximetry is a continuous, noninvasive method for monitoring the patient's arterial oxygen saturation. It is an early indicator of hypoxemia. Oxygen is typically administered via nasal cannula, which is always placed before the medication administration. Explanation of the monitoring devices and the sounds the patient will encounter will allay patient anxiety. Intravenous (IV) access is then obtained (20-gauge or larger catheter in adult populations or per hospital policy). The IV access provides a means of delivering conscious sedation medications and implementing emergency medications, fluids, and reversal agents in the instance of an untoward event.

Patient exposure during the procedure is another nursing responsibility. The patient must be exposed appropriately while maintaining normothermia. Keeping the environmental temperature and length of time the patient will be exposed are important points to keep in mind. Maintaining ambient temperature and applying warm blankets preserves normothermia.

Patient Positioning

Depending on the procedure, the patient is assisted to the appropriate position needed. It is the nurse's responsibility to assure that bony prominences and pressure points are padded to prevent injury. The nurse should take a proactive attitude in providing patient safety and protection from injury. The patient should be in as comfortable a position as possible without undue flexion, extension, or compression of any extremity to prevent nerve injury. Brachial plexus injury can occur easily due to the superficial nature of this nerve bundle along the axilla. Avoiding abduction of the arm greater than 90° while the head is turned toward the opposite direction can prevent this occurrence. The lithotomy position has the potential for damaging several nerves by excessive thigh flexion or angulation. Compression due to the stirrups or lithotomy knee brace used also may effect nerve compression. Furthermore, the patient's skin must be protected from irritation secondary to improperly grounded electrical equipment used, friction, or pressure. Many of the procedures using conscious sedation have formerly been preformed in the operating room. Hence, many of the same issues in the operating room area are relevant even in brief, outpatient scenarios.

Patient position also effects pulmonary function. A patient with obstructive or restrictive pulmonary disease may lose up to 1.0 liter of functional residual capacity in the supine position, decreasing the pulmonary reserve. The patient with pulmonary disease may also have a decreased arterial oxygen level (pO_2) and/or increase carbon dioxide level (pCO_2). These physiologic factors coupled with the administration of sedating medication may call for more intensive monitoring and/or environment. Smoking history, pulmonary function tests, and baseline arterial blood gas values will assist the physician in decision making about conscious sedation medications and environment. Oxygen must always be applied prior to medication administration.

During the Procedure

The nurse's main responsibilities during the delivery of conscious sedation are patient monitoring and assessment and treatment of untoward responses to therapy.

Monitoring and Assessment

As a general guideline, the nurse monitoring the patient receiving conscious sedation should have no other responsibilities than that patient's care. This issue has been revisited many times in the intensive care unit (ICU) setting, where nurses often are assigned two patients. If conscious sedation is being administered to an ICU patient, that nurse should temporarily relinquish care of the second patient to another qualified health care provider (nurse or physician). It is the responsibility of the institution to assure safe and appropriate nurse staffing. Once the patient receiving conscious sedation has recovered from the procedure, the nurse may resume care of the second patient. The rationale for these preventative measures is well founded. Potential for acute hemodynamic and ventilatory compromise is inherent to conscious sedation. Therefore, continuous monitoring of vital signs, oxygenation, and level of sedation is paramount and having other responsibilities could compromise care during the procedure.

The question of how often to monitor a patient's vital signs depends on established institutional guidelines. A baseline set of vital signs should be obtained and used for comparison throughout the procedure. Once medications are administered, full sets of vital signs should be documented every 5 minutes or more often as indicated by patient status. A complete set of vital signs includes cardiac rhythm and rate, respiratory rate, oxygen saturation, blood pressure, level of consciousness, and skin signs. Typically, IV access is maintained with an isotonic solution to keep the vein open and increased as needed to deliver medications. The patient's response to the procedure and medications must be carefully documented.

The key to successful patient care during conscious sedation is continuous monitoring and assessment. The patient's airway patency, gas exchange, level of consciousness, and hemodynamic response to therapies all require advanced nursing skill and assessment. The nurse must further assess whether the patient is receiving adequate analgesia and anxiolysis versus oversedation.

Medication Administration

The nurse or physician may administer conscious sedation medications. The attending physician prescribes medications based on many factors. These factors include the patient's age, weight, allergies, and previous reaction to pain-relieving and sedating medications. Personal preference for the combination of medications is based on several aspects. These include previous experience with administering a particular drug, its cost, and the length of the procedure. Standard combinations of medications may be adopted and implemented in institutional guidelines or procedures. However, there is no standard dose of any particular medication for a given procedure. Drug dosing is a highly individualized task based on many medical judgments. There is a fine line between light and deep sedation; therefore, medications must be titrated slowly and according to patient response. Crossing the line into deep sedation may necessitate intubation and resuscitation. The physician must be present when the medications are administered and remain present until the procedure is complete. An IV access and oxygen delivery device (usually a nasal cannula) must be in place prior to medication administration.

There are four categories of commonly prescribed medications. These include opioids (morphine, fentanyl), benzodiazepines (midazolam, lorazepam), IV anesthetics (propofol, ketamine), and hypnotics/CNS depressants (pentobarbital) (see Chapter 1). The nurse is responsible for understanding the rationale for administering medications, their pharmacology, side effects (both desirable and undesirable), and interactions, including the use of reversal agents.

TABLE 2. Checklist for the RN Managing Patients Receiving Conscious Sedation

❏   The physician is present

❏   IV access is maintained at all times

❏   Monitoring equipment is in place—vital signs every 5 minutes and PRN

❏   Supplemental oxygen is immediately available

❏   Emergency cart with defibrillator is immediately accessible

Managing Complications

The main complications that patients experience include oversedation, respiratory depression, cardiac arrhythmias, and hemodynamic instability. Treatment of these complications and use of reversal agents should be a topic of training prior to staff caring for patient receiving conscious sedation. Abnormal vital signs must be acted upon swiftly and properly. This requires knowledge of the function and proper use of monitoring and emergency equipment. Skills needed to appropriately treat emergencies include CPR, basic airway management, oxygen delivery systems, defibrillation, cardiac arrhythmia interpretation, and parenteral fluid administration. Additional assistance should be summoned at once (depending on environment).

In treating complications, it is important for the nurse to revert to the ABCs. Maintaining airway patency is vital. The airway may become blocked due to the patient's tongue, secretions, or head position. The nurse should immediately reposition the patient's head and clear the airway. Suction may be necessary to clear secretions and prevent aspirations. Insert an oral or nasopharyngeal airway if needed. Sometimes the stimulation of clearing the airway and repositioning the head is enough to confirm a patent airway. The patient should respond to verbal command as well, unless oversedated. If these measures do not adequately treat the problem, provide increased stimulation and encourage the patient to take deep breaths. Assess the patient's respiratory rate, depth, use of respiratory musculature, and oxygen saturation. If they are inadequate, apply positive-pressure ventilation via bag-valve mask. A few minutes of assisted breathing may improve the situation.

Vital signs often may vary 10–20% from the baseline once conscious sedation medications are given. Any decrease greater than 20% from baseline should

TABLE 3. Return to Preprocedure Function[2]

Return of preprocedure level of consciousness
Adequate respiratory function
Absence of significant pain
Stable vital signs
Absence of nausea
Satisfactory surgical site and dressing condition (if present)
Intact protective reflexes
Normal skin color and condition
Return of preprocedure motor and sensory control
Normothermia

be taken very seriously. Simple hypotension that lasts for more than a few minutes may be treated with a fluid bolus (often 250–500 ml 0.9% normal saline) without patient compromise. This, of course, requires a doctor's order. A persistent hypotension of greater than 20% from baseline should be treated more aggressively. The nurse should investigate the cause of the hypotension, consider reversal agents, and even vasopressors (dopamine or phenylephrine).

Hypertension also may occur and is most often due to inadequate pain or anxiety control. Assess the patient's level of consciousness and any signs of pain (e.g., grimacing). An additional dose of pain or anxiety-relieving medication may be indicated.

Patients may experience cardiac arrhythmias as a result of the procedure or medications received during conscious sedation. Although bradycardia and tachycardia are the most common arrhythmias seen, there is a potential for other arrhythmias such as ventricular ectopy and atrial arrhythmias (atrial fibrillation). Bradycardia is caused by vagal stimulation (during endoscopy) and hypoxia. Tachycardia can result from inadequate sedation, pain, and hypotension. Intravenous fluid and/or increased sedation can provide a return to a normal heart rate and rhythm. If these interventions are not successful, assess the patient for another cause of arrhythmia. In cases of undetermined arrhythmia or when ST-segment changes are noted, a 12-lead EKG should be obtained for further diagnosis and treatment. Complex arrhythmias should be treated as indicated (antiarrhythmic agents, resuscitative measures, and defibrillation). Because of the potential for these arrhythmias, ACLS certification is recommended for all health care providers administering conscious sedation.

When untoward events take place, the health care providers must be in agreement whether or not to continue the procedure. The options include continuing the procedure or aborting the procedure with or without use of reversal agents. Need for further resuscitative measures would preclude continuing the procedure. It is important for the team to agree on the safest treatment plan.

After the Procedure

Recovery

At the conclusion of the procedure, the patient must be monitored for a specified amount of time. The amount of time for recovery is subject to institutional and practice standards. This time depends on the type and length of the procedure as well as the patient's response to medications administered. Vital signs are usually documented at least every 15 minutes. The patient is monitored for return of preprocedure function and vital signs (Table 3).

Discharge and Patient Education

Standard discharge criteria must be specified in institutional guidelines. These criteria should be developed by a multidisciplinary team that includes members of anesthesia, medical, and nursing team and other departments as appropriate. It is mandatory that the patient be discharged to a responsible adult. They should be instructed on postprocedure care, expectations (pain control, amnesia of the event), and follow-up. Due to the frequency of decreased memory following conscious sedation, all instructions should be given in writing to the adult escort. The patient should be able to return to activities of daily living upon discharge. Patients who do not meet discharge criteria should remain monitored until their preprocedure function has returned.

Specific teaching for self-care of affected areas and activity limitations (driving, heavy lifting, exercise, etc.) should be clearly understood. For example, patients with minor operative procedures should be able to take care of the incision and should avoid lifting anything heavy for 2 weeks. The patient must be instructed not to drive, use alcohol, or make important decisions for the next 24 hours as there are residual effects of the medications. The potential for complications such as infection must be discussed before the patient leaves. They must be instructed what signs and symptoms they should look for (fever, redness, swelling, odor, pain, bleeding, drainage) and when to call the doctor. The doctor's phone number and information about a follow-up appointment should be included in their written discharge instructions.

Documentation

Complete and accurate documentation of the conscious sedation procedure is essential. A single form that encompasses the entire conscious sedation procedure, from preprocedure through recovery, may be used. Documentation may be divided into several segments. The first segment includes, but is not limited to, the pre-procedure assessment, history, vital signs, ASA classification and Mallampati score. The second segment includes the medications and fluids used, physiologic data, intraprocedure events, level of consciousness, equipment used, and nursing interventions taken. After medications and nursing interventions are administered, the patient's response to the intervention must be documented. The time, dose, and route of medications must be clearly noted. Rating systems such as the Ramsey scale are often helpful in providing descriptors of patient responses to sedating medications. Other rating scales for pain such as the visual analog scale or a 1–10 scale may be used when the patient is fully awake. Patient response to interventions and medications must be described in the charting. The final section allows space to document recovery vital signs, level of consciousness, and assessment of the patient's return to normal function. A single form that may be used by multiple disciplines (nursing, medicine, respiratory) is ideal. It is advisable to use a conscious sedation form when conscious sedation is administered in the intensive care unit. Most currently used ICU flow sheets do not provide adequate space for completely documenting the events taking place during a conscious sedation procedure. Some facilities have gone to computerized charting systems, which allow for documenting vital signs every 5 minutes and provide ample room for multiple disciplines to chart. An example of such a form is provided (Fig. 1).

Legal Issues

Authority for registered nurses to administer medications is derived from each state's Nurse Practice Act. Each state's Board of Registered Nursing administers the Nurse Practice Act. It is this body that determines whether certain activities are within the legal realm of the state's Nurse Practice Act. No state Nurse Practice Act addresses the issue of monitoring of patients receiving conscious sedation. However, many states have issued their own position statements regarding the nurse's role in conscious sedation procedures. In many cases, the position statement defines the concept, environmental requirements and circumstances under which the registered nurse may be involved in delivery of conscious sedation. The position statement may also serve to clarify the difference in roles between a registered nurse and certified registered nurse anesthetist (CRNA). This might include circumstances in which specific drugs may not be used, as they are defined within the CRNA domain. Nurses should look up their respective Board of Registered Nursing and Practice Act to verify that administration of conscious sedation is within the scope of their practice.

It must be emphasized that the monitoring of patients receiving conscious sedation is not a basic nursing skill. Advanced knowledge and skills are required to safely care for patients receiving conscious sedation. Because of this, even if

CONSCIOUS SEDATION RECORD

UNIT NUMBER:

PATIENT NAME:

DATE OF BIRTH:

LOCATION: DATE:

DATE: _____ PROCEDURE _____

Time of last PO intake   Solids: _____   Fluids: _____   ☐ Consent signed: ☐ H&P in chart

☐ Ride home available   ☐ Ride home, not applicable   Allergies   ☐ NKA ☐ Yes: _____

MONITORING EQUIPMENT   ☐ Non-invasive BP   ☐ Pulse oximeter   ☐ ECG/alarms on   ☐ O$_2$ _____ l/min

☐ Emergency supplies (resuscitation, equipment, suction, reversal agents available)   ☐ Venous access

☐ ID banc ☐ Pre-procedure teaching completed/understood   ☐ Baseline level of consciousness _____

PRE-PROCEDURE NOTE: ☐ Risks, benefits, and alternatives of the procedure and risks and options of conscious sedation explained to patient.

Plan for sedation: ☐ IV sedation with _____

☐ Other: _____

Date: _____ MD signature _____ ID # _____

PROCEDURE TIME			MONITORING	Comments
Start:	Finish	Time / Baseline / / / / / / / / / / / / / / / Time		

Local Anesthetic Agent

MONT ☐
O$_2$ ☐   200, 180
BP v ^   160, 140
PULSE ●   120, 100
TEMP △   80
RESP ○   60, 40
          20

Time	Medication	Amount	Route

SpO$_2$

Sedation Level

Tolerance to Procedure

IV Solution	Amount absorbed
Total:	

POST-PROCEDURE NOTE:

☐ Patient meets recovery criteria   ☐ Orders written for continued monitoring upon transfer to unit

Time _____ MD signature _____ ID # _____

Patient disposition to: ☐ Home with responsible adult ☐ Home AMA ☐ Other _____ ☐ Inpatient unit ____ ☐ PACU ☐ Other _____

RN signature _____ Time _____

	Sedation Level Criteria	score	Tolerance to Procedure Criteria	score	Recovery Criteria
KEY	Fully awake and oriented	1	Pain/discomfort absent	1	Vital signs stable and returned to baseline
	Drowsy and anxiety free	2	Pain/discomfort moderate to distressing	2	Level of consciousness back to baseline
	Easily arousable to verbal stimuli	3	Severe discomfort	3	Oxygen saturation ≥ 95% or baseline
	Eyes closed, arousable to mild stimulation	4			Stable cardiovascular status
	Eyes closed, unresponsive to mild stimulation	5			Able to transport home with responsible adult

CONSCIOUS SEDATION RECORD

Figure 1. Sample documentation sheet for conscious sedation.

conscious sedation is a clearly accepted nursing action by a particular state, nurses who assume this endeavor need additional training and education. Many states directly refer to position statements of nursing professional organizations, such as the Association of Operating Room Nurses (AORN), American Nurses Association (ANA), or the American Association of Nurse Anesthetists (AANA). These organizations' position statements provide a reference for standard of care on a national level and are influential in effecting policy changes.

Institutional Policies and Guidelines

Most position statements from both the state and organizational level specify that institutions have policies or guidelines in place that define and evaluate the nurse's role in providing conscious sedation. The nurse's competence in this task should be documented on a periodic basis. The Joint Commission on Accreditation of Healthcare Organizations (JCAHO) also has taken a role in determining national performance standards for delivery of conscious sedation. JCAHO is an independent, not-for-profit organization that evaluates quality and performance standards in health care organizations nationwide. One of its areas of activity is assessing an institution's standard of care and performance outcomes. If the institution complies with JCAHO mandates, it usually results in good patient outcomes.

JCAHO has paid special attention to this issue because of the inherent difficulty in predicting patient responses to conscious sedation. Per JCAHO, a hospital must have a conscious sedation program. Noncompliance with JCAHO standards can result in a type I recommendation: "A type I recommendation requires the health care organization to resolve insufficient or unsatisfactory standards compliance in a specific performance area. The organization must resolve type I recommendations in a specified amount of time to maintain its accreditation."[4] Loss of accreditation can ultimately lead to loss of revenue to the institution in a variety of ways, thus it is important to the institution to have a conscious sedation program that complies with JCAHO standards. JCAHO compliance maintains a certain standard of care, improves patient outcomes, decreases patient risk, and helps secure institution funding. It is good practice to consult the JCAHO manual when developing a policy and procedure regarding conscious sedation.

According to JCAHO, an institutional policy or guidelines must encompass the following five areas:
1. Sufficient personnel to perform the procedure
2. Appropriate equipment for care and resuscitation
3. Appropriate monitoring of vital signs
4. Appropriate documentation of care
5. Monitoring of outcomes[4]

The policy should clearly identify what drugs and doses are standard in the institution's use, patient assessment, criteria for NPO status, documentation, discharge criteria, and establishing staff competence and training.

The institutional guidelines for administering and monitoring conscious sedation should apply uniformly in all settings. The basic principles of the conscious sedation policy and competence apply to its administration regardless of where the nurse is employed (endoscopy suite, cardiac catheterization lab, emergency room, etc.). However, unit-specific (e.g., pediatric or geriatric) needs may be added to baseline skills and knowledge.

Education and Validation of Competence

The registered nurse caring for the patient receiving conscious sedation must be clinically competent in that responsibility. Evidence of this competence should be established through a competence-based training program and reevaluated on a periodic basis. Knowledge of anatomy, physiology, pharmacology of conscious sedation medications, cardiac rhythm interpretation, and respiratory function provide the theoretical foundation for subsequent nursing practice. An understanding of these concepts bestows the rationale for possible complications of conscious sedation and their management. To act correctly and provide safe care, the nurse must understand how to operate monitoring and resuscitation equipment. This includes the automatic vital sign monitors, airway devices (bag-valve mask, airway adjuncts), oxygen delivery equipment, cardiac monitor, defibrillator, suction apparatus, and IV supplies. Basic and advanced cardiac life support (BLS and ACLS) certification or their equivalents must be a portion of the competence-based program. Rapid intervention is needed in the event of complications. The nurse should have a variety of basic and advanced skills in order to ensure for optimal patient outcomes.

To assure an adequately trained staff, the institution should provide the means to guarantee a basic level of training for all staff members involved in the delivery of conscious sedation. Components of the training should include a variety of teaching methodologies that are geared for adult learners. Providing verbal, written, and interactive approaches will yield the highest level of compliance and retention of material from involved staff. Institutional requirements may overlap with those of conscious sedation (BLS, ACLS, and airway management).

The program should include some form of didactic. Exact descriptions of skills and knowledge should be provided prior to training to enhance student success and decrease misconceptions. This can be achieved by using a study module, lectures, or videos. Content knowledge such as anatomy and pharmacology can be established with a written exam. This may be provided before formal training to assess baseline knowledge or at the end of a training program to evaluate student learning. Hands-on instruction and role-playing are other teaching strategies that foster motor performance of skills.

In competence-based training, evaluating nurses' knowledge and behavior is the goal to establishing competence. A checklist of relevant skills and behaviors (including use of equipment) with criteria for successful completion is used for evaluation of the learner in the practice environment. Observation by a senior staff nurse and/or nurse educator in the practice environment using the performance checklist provides for establishing behavioral competence.

Conclusion

In light of an ever-changing health care environment, safe and skillful delivery of conscious sedation is of utmost importance to all members of the health care team. Nurses play an important and unique role in successful outcomes. Rarely, if ever, does conscious sedation take place without a registered nurse present. They are most often the primary caregiver before, during, and after the procedure. They are the patient advocate and educator, while all the time providing emotional and spiritual support. Thus, nurses have a role and obligation in developing and influencing state and organizational practice guidelines for conscious sedation.

References

1. American Association of Critical Care Nurses: Position Statement—Role of the RN in Conscious Sedation, 1996. Available online at: http://www.aacn.org/aacn/practice
2. American Society of Anesthesiologists: The ASA physical status classification system, 1999. Available online at: http://www.asahq.org/ProfInfo/PhysicalStatus.html
3. Association of Operating Room Nurses (AORN) Board of Directors: Recommended practices for managing the patient receiving conscious sedation/analgesia. AORN J 65: 129–134, 1997.
4. Joint Commission on Accreditation of Healthcare Organizations, 1999. Available online at the JCAHO home page: http://wwwb.jcaho.org/sentinel/type1.html
5. Mallampati SR, Gatt SP, Gugino LD, et al: A clinical sign to predict difficult tracheal intubation: A prospective study. Can Anaesth Soc J 32:429–434, 1985.
6. Watson DS, James DS: Intravenous conscious sedation: Implications of monitoring patients receiving local anesthesia. AORN J 51:1512–1522, 1990.

12

Legal Issues in Conscious Sedation

Richard J. Kelly, M.D., J.D., M.P.H.

With the advent of short-acting anesthetic drugs and the development of minimally invasive surgical techniques, minor surgeries once performed in the operating room may now be performed under conscious sedation in other areas of the hospital and in outpatient surgery centers. The cost savings realized by outpatient surgeries have created a very strong trend away from operating room use. If this trend continues, outpatient surgeries may account for up to 82% of the total surgical volume in the U.S. by the year 2005, with a significant increase in the use of conscious sedation.

Although the delivery of conscious sedation no longer requires the knowledge and skill of a qualified anesthesiologist, it is not without potential risks for medical malpractice liability. Regardless of the quality of care provided, unanticipated complications occur during conscious sedation that may have dramatic adverse consequences for the patient. When these undesirable complications lead to malpractice litigation, the physician must understand the legal process and be prepared to convince the court that his or her actions were within the standard of care for the profession.

This chapter focuses on the elements of professional liability with a discussion of the applicable standard of care for conscious sedation. It also reviews actions that may be taken to minimize the risk of medical malpractice when delivering conscious sedation and the manner in which a potential lawsuit should be addressed.

Professional Liability

When a complication occurs during the delivery of conscious sedation, the patient or the patient's heirs may choose to sue the physician based on the legal theory of professional negligence. To prevail in the suit, the plaintiff must prove each of the four elements of professional negligence: (1) the physician owed to the patient a duty; (2) the physician failed in his duty to the patient; (3) a close causal relationship exists between the physician's actions and the patient's injury; and (4) the patient suffered actual damage or injury due to the physician's breach of the standard of care. All four elements must be proved or the negligence suit will fail.

Duty

When a physician sees a patient preoperatively and agrees to provide conscious sedation or any other medical service, the physician is establishing a duty to the patient. The duty the physician owes to the patient is to treat the patient with the same standard of care as would be rendered by a reasonable and prudent physician in the same or similar circumstances.

One of the first duties the physician has toward the patient is to obtain the patient's informed consent to proceed with the conscious sedation. In order to properly obtain informed consent, the physician must explain the proposed conscious sedation to the patient in sufficient detail so that the patient may make an informed decision whether to proceed or refuse to undergo conscious sedation. The failure of the physician to fulfill this duty can subject the physician to charges of battery.

Breach of Duty

If the patient pursues a civil action for medical malpractice based on negligence, the patient must prove that the physician did something that should not have been done or did not do something that should have been done and, in so doing, failed to adhere to the standard of care of a reasonable and prudent physician. Usually the patient's attorney will retain a qualified medical expert to review the medical records and determine whether, in the opinion of the expert, the physician's actions fell below the applicable standard of care.

Causation

The breach of the physician's duty of care must be related to the injury or damage the patient suffered. If a physician breached his duty of care but the patient suffered no injury as a result, the element of causation will fail. Likewise, if the physician's actions fell below the standard of care and the patient was injured but the injury was not related to the physician's failure to maintain the standard of care, the causation element also will fail. Only when the physician's actions fell below the standard of care and those same actions were the proximate cause of the patient's injury will this element of causation be met.

The burden to prove causation usually is the responsibility of the plaintiff, but in the case of conscious sedation, where drugs are administered that may render the patient amnesic, the burden of proof may be shifted to the physician under the doctrine of *res ipsa loquitur* (Latin for "the thing speaks for itself"). The doctrine requires the plaintiff to prove the following in order to shift the burden of proof to the defendant: (1) the injury suffered by the plaintiff would not occur in the absence of negligence; (2) the injury was caused by something under the exclusive control of the physician; (3) the patient did not contribute in any way to the injury; and (4) the physician has more accessibility to the evidence to explain the events than does the patient. If these four conditions of the res ipsa loquitor doctrine are satisfied, the plaintiff is relieved of the burden of proving causation and the burden is shifted to the defendant to prove that he or she was not negligent.

Damages

The fourth element of a cause of action for negligence is showing that the patient suffered actual damage as a result of the breach of the standard of care. The plaintiff can claim three different kinds of damages. The first, general damages, is the pain and suffering that was a direct result of the injury. The second, special damages, is the actual monetary damages that occurred as a result of the injury. These may include additional hospital bills, lost wages, and additional expenditures to accommodate the injury. The third kind of damages, which usually do not apply to professional negligence, is the punitive damages that are assessed to punish the physician for negligence that was particularly egregious, reckless, or deliberate. The dollar amount of the damages is usually decided by the jury, taking into account the difference between the patient's present condition and the condition he would have been in if the negligence had not occurred.

Standard of Care for Conscious Sedation

In a cause of action for professional negligence, the attorneys for each party usually retain a medical expert to establish the applicable standard of care. In the past, these expert witnesses described for the court what they believed to be the standard of care for the community. Federal regulations of health care delivery and managed care, however, have all but eliminated regional standards of care in favor of national standards.

The Joint Commission on Accreditation of Healthcare Organizations (JCAHO) is the federal body that, through its accreditation process, establishes the standard of care for medical procedures in health care organizations throughout the United States. The JCAHO standards do not directly address the administration of conscious sedation, but the current position of the JCAHO is that the standards of care for general anesthesia should apply to all patients undergoing any kind of anesthesia, including conscious sedation, in all areas of the hospital and in outpatient settings.

A general consensus has emerged from recent JCAHO hearings that the current standards for the delivery of anesthesia no longer reflect changes that have occurred in clinical anesthesia in recent years and, as a result, the JCAHO has begun the process of redefining its standards for anesthesia care. The Standards and Survey Procedures Committee of the JCAHO has been authorized to develop new standards for anesthesia procedures, including conscious sedation, using definitions approved by the American Society of Anesthesiologists. The new JCAHO conscious sedation standards are expected to be approved in the near future.

In response to the need for national standards of care for conscious sedation, medical organizations such as the American Society of Anesthesiologists, the American Nurses Association, and the American Dental Association have developed practice standards that may serve as guides to acceptable clinical practice for their respective professions. These guidelines define a standard of care for conscious sedation that will minimize the risks associated with conscious sedation but allow physicians and dentists the flexibility to tailor their anesthetics to fit the surgical procedure and the medical status of the patient. In many instances, these practice guidelines are based on research of the applicable literature and therefore should be considered the minimum requirements for sound clinical practice.

A minority of states have laws that regulate the use of conscious sedation. Most of these states have used the guidelines of one of the national professional organizations as a template for their legislation. Some states, however, have included more detailed requirements such as the qualifications of support personnel, mandatory reporting of adverse events, and adequacy of the anesthesia equipment. Physicians and other health care personnel should adhere closely to the requirements of their own state laws. In those jurisdictions where the delivery of conscious sedation is not regulated by state law, physicians would be well served by following the practice guidelines that have been developed by their national organization.

Definition of Conscious Sedation

Conscious sedation, which represents only one portion of the continuum between full consciousness and complete obtundation, has been variably defined by the national professional organizations and states legislatures. Physicians, dentists, and nurses should clearly understand the parameters of conscious sedation for their state and their profession to avoid the danger of liability that may arise from practicing outside of these definitions of conscious sedation.

According to the American Nurses Association, "a patient under conscious sedation has a depressed level of consciousness, but retains the ability to independently and continuously maintain a patent airway and respond appropriately to physical stimulation and/or verbal command."

The American Dental Association (ADA) defines conscious sedation as "a minimally depressed level of consciousness that retains the patient's ability to independently and continuously maintain an airway and respond appropriately to physical stimulation or verbal command." The ADA definition for conscious sedation also states that patients are no longer consciously sedated if they only reflexively withdraw from "repeated" painful stimuli.

The American Society of Anesthesiologists (ASA) has abandoned the term conscious sedation in favor of the term sedation and analgesia to describe the state of consciousness that "allows patients to tolerate unpleasant procedures while maintaining adequate cardiorespiratory function and the ability to respond purposefully to verbal command and/or tactile stimulation." The ASA also notes that "patients whose only response is reflex withdrawal from a painful stimulus are sedated to a greater degree than encompassed by sedation/analgesia."

The term "monitored anesthesia care" is not synonymous with conscious sedation and differs in two important respects. First, a patient under conscious sedation, by definition, must maintain spontaneous breathing and purposeful responses throughout the procedure. Monitored anesthesia care, on the other hand, may include conscious sedation but it also allows the physician to administer anesthetic drugs that cause both a loss of consciousness and loss of protective airway reflexes. Second, conscious sedation may be administered by a nurse or other qualified person under the supervision of a physician or dentist, while monitored anesthesia care requires the continuous presence of a physician whose sole responsibility is to monitor the patient.

Qualifications to Administer Conscious Sedation

In general, physicians, nurses, and dentists should consult their own hospital's credentials committee to determine whether they are qualified to administer conscious sedation. Hospital credentials committees ensure that their staff are in compliance with JCAHO and state law requirements by incorporating these requirements into the hospital's own requirements for administering conscious sedation.

However, since the JCAHO currently has no published standard of care for the delivery of conscious sedation, the Joint Commission recommends that competence criteria for the administration of conscious sedation be included in the competency criteria for the procedures that use conscious sedation. Thus, a physician who applies to have privileges to perform endoscopies at his hospital must have the appropriate education, training, and experience not only to safely perform endoscopies but also to administer the conscious sedation.

State laws generally do not specify the qualifications needed for physicians to administer conscious sedation other than to require that physicians possess valid medical licenses to practice in the state and satisfy the hospital's requirements (and thus the JCAHO's requirements) for certification to perform conscious sedation.

As a practical matter, hospitals should require physicians who wish to perform or supervise the administration of conscious sedation to have, at a minimum, current ACLS certification and documentation that they either have successfully managed a sufficient number of cases in the past several years or have the requisite education and training to administer conscious sedation.

Registered nurses may be asked by a physician or dentist to administer drugs to achieve conscious sedation. The American Nurses Association recommends that nurses who administer the drugs not only have the appropriate qualifications as defined by state law and hospital policy but also possess the requisite education to understand the pharmacology of the drugs, the physiology that accompanies conscious sedation, and the ability to recognize and treat cardiopulmonary complications.

Risk Management

Adequate educational preparation and experience, while necessary, is not by itself sufficient to ensure the safe and effective use of conscious sedation. There is always some degree of risk associated with the use of any drug even when administered by trained individuals. Health care professionals who are certified to use conscious sedation should take the following important steps to ensure the safety of the patient and minimize liability.

Patient Selection

Physicians will minimize their exposure to risk by the realization that not all patients are necessarily appropriate candidates for conscious sedation. Preverbal children, the elderly, and patients with unusually high anxiety generally should be considered poor candidates for conscious sedation.

Preverbal children lack the ability to consistently respond purposefully to commands and assessing their level of consciousness may prove difficult. If these children do obstruct their airways, they will desaturate, become bradycardic, and experience cardiac arrest much more quickly than a healthy adult.

Elderly patients should be considered poor candidates for conscious sedation for very different reasons. The elderly tend to respond to sedative drugs with vastly different pharmacodynamic and pharmacokinetic profiles that may make predicting their responses to medications much more difficult. Some elderly patients will develop paradoxical excitation with increasing doses of sedative drugs, while others may achieve deep sedation or, worse, apnea with only minute doses. Also, the chance of encountering an adverse drug reaction under conscious sedation increases with the elderly who tend to ingest more over-the-counter and prescription medications than the general population.

Conscious sedation is best used for the management of mild anxiety. Patients with greater than mild anxiety or patients who previously have been uncooperative under conscious sedation are not good candidates for conscious sedation because they may require increasingly larger doses of sedative drugs to assure their cooperation. These large doses of sedative medication may lead to an increased risk of airway obstruction, apnea, and anoxic brain injury.

Physicians do not necessarily need to categorically eliminate preverbal children, the elderly, or very anxious patients from receiving conscious sedation but these patients should be screened carefully to prevent the need to handle untoward complications in a setting that may not be equipped to handle such complications.

Preanesthetic Evaluation

The purpose of the preanesthetic evaluation is to identify patients who might experience complications during or after the administration of sedative medications. Physicians and dentists should choose only patients who are likely to benefit from conscious sedation and exclude patients who may be at high risk or in need of further evaluation.

A physician who identifies severe but treatable medical problems during the preanesthetic evaluation should delay the surgical procedure and request that the patient undergo further medical evaluation. Physicians should not feel pressured to provide conscious sedation against their better judgment and risk a possible adverse outcomes simply to keep up with busy surgical schedules. Physicians who succumb to such pressure may be hard pressed to explain in a court of law why conscious sedation was administered for an elective procedure when further work-up or treatment may have made the procedure safer. Altogether, restricting the use of conscious sedation to patients who are appropriate candidates will limit the incidence of adverse outcomes, increase rates of patient satisfaction, and reduce liability exposure.

Informed Consent

Physicians are required by law in virtually every state of the nation to obtain informed consent from their patients before subjecting them to any treatment or procedure. The intent of the informed consent doctrine is to provide patients with sufficient information to allow them to participate in their own health care decisions. In this regard, patients should be informed that the administration of conscious sedation may pose risks that are independent of, and sometimes exceeding, the risks of the actual surgical procedure. After considering the information presented to them, competent patients have the right to accept or refuse the care offered, and physicians who proceed with conscious sedation without consent may be found liable for battery.

Occasionally, physicians are confronted with patients who attempt to withdraw their informed consent during the surgical procedure due to increased anxiety or discomfort. The law is clear that competent patients may withdraw their informed consent to a procedure or treatment at any time. Patients who have already received sedative or analgesic medications, however, may no longer be considered competent either to give additional informed consent or withdraw their informed consent for the procedure. In cases in which the patient requests that the procedure be terminated, the physician should seek continued informed consent from a person who may act as a surrogate for the patient, such as the next of kin or the person holding the patient's durable power of attorney for health care. In the absence of a surrogate, the physician must use his or her best judgment whether to continue or abort the procedure, taking into account the patient's state of mind prior to the procedure, the discomfort of the patient, the ability to abort the procedure, and the diagnostic and therapeutic importance of the procedure. If possible, the physician should seek the advice of a risk manager in the hospital if such a person is readily available.

To shield themselves from liability, physicians should document all informed consent discussions. This documentation should include the content of the disclosure, evidence of the patient's understanding, the presence of translation services, if needed, and the patient's consent to undergo the procedure.

Personnel

The physician should ensure that there are enough qualified personnel present to perform the procedure and monitor the patient. Since the physician is responsible for performing the surgical procedure and must concentrate on the task at hand, there should be at least one other designated, qualified individual exclusively assigned to administer sedative drugs and monitor the patient. The individual managing the anesthetic care of the patient ideally should have no other responsibilities that would leave the patient unattended or compromise continuous monitoring. The presence of an adequate number of qualified personnel will reduce the chance that a dangerous condition such as apnea or an abnormal cardiac rhythm is overlooked. When an adverse event does occur, the presence of additional qualified personnel may help stabilize the situation more quickly.

Drugs

Careful selection of sedative drugs is the cornerstone of a safe conscious sedation. To reduce the chance of malpractice liability, physicians should studiously avoid using a single combination of drugs with the same dosages for every patient. Patients vary dramatically in their responsiveness to sedative drugs and it should not be assumed that there is any universally safe and effective dosing regimen for achieving conscious sedation in all patients. Instead, physicians should consider each patient's anesthetic requirements carefully and select drugs that carry a wide margin of safety and for which the unintended loss of consciousness is highly unlikely. In choosing the drug regimen for a particular patient, the practitioner should consider his or her own familiarity with the drugs, the medical condition of the patient, the appropriateness of the facility to handle adverse effects of the drugs, and the availability of trained personnel to assist in the management of emergent situations.

Drugs for conscious sedation usually work well for healthy patients with mild anxiety. On occasion, patients may become uncooperative as they become sedated. In these situations, it is wiser to apologize for some discomfort during a procedure or halt the procedure altogether rather than deepening the sedation in an attempt to gain the patient's cooperation and risk the possibility of causing airway complications in what might otherwise be a minor procedure.

Sometimes, despite careful titration of sedative drugs, patients may become more deeply sedated than anticipated and have respiratory compromise or loss of airway reflexes. The amount of training, experience, and skill needed to safely manage central nervous system depression increases as the degree with which the patient is sedated increases. In these cases where the degree of sedation is higher than anticipated, an anesthesiologist or nurse anesthetist should be summoned. If such help is not immediately available, the procedure should be abandoned and attention should be directed toward maintaining the patient's airway and administering drugs that will reverse the sedative effects. Again, it is wiser to halt the procedure altogether than to risk liability for undesired complications.

Monitoring the Patient

The person trained in conscious sedation who is managing the care of the patient should continuously monitor the patient from the onset of conscious sedation through recovery. This person should record the patient's condition at regular intervals and be able to recognize airway obstruction and adverse drug reactions as well as respond to trends in respiratory rate, pulse oximetry, blood pressure, heart rate, and level of consciousness for the duration of the conscious sedation.

The person managing the conscious sedation should have present and in use all of the monitoring equipment necessary for conscious sedation. This person should also have established IV access for rapid administration of drugs and have the ability to summon additional help if needed. Since the duration of the effects of anesthesia medications can persist after the completion of the procedure, monitoring should continue until the patient achieves the criteria for discharge.

Documentation

Be certain to document fully. The medical record is the foundation upon which a medical malpractice defense is built. When information is missing from the medical record, the plaintiff in the malpractice action may raise questions whether certain actions were actually performed and cast doubt about the motives of the person who failed to record the information. It is absolutely imperative to document all essential information carefully and completely even in situations in which potential liability is not anticipated.

At a minimum, the anesthetic chart for conscious sedation should contain documentation that the heart rate, blood pressure, respiratory rate, and responsiveness of the patient were checked at specific, regular intervals. The documentation of care should begin at the time the physician or dentist initiates the induction for conscious sedation and should continue until the time the patient has recovered from the sedation. For conscious sedation in critical care units, the documentation can be charted on the unit flow sheet. Otherwise, the documentation for patients receiving conscious sedation should be done on an approved conscious sedation record.

Criteria for Discharge

Discharging patients who are still under the influence of sedative drugs has been the basis for several medical negligence lawsuits. Those patients were discharged prematurely, had airway compromise, aspirated, and died in the car on the way home or required admission to the intensive care unit. It is absolutely essential that the responsible physician be certain that the patient is awake, alert, able to sit up unaided and, if not limited by any other medical condition, able to ambulate without assistance prior to discharge. Upon discharge, the patient and a family member should be given written and verbal care instructions as well as a 24-hour emergency telephone number to call for any questions or concerns. Ideally, the patient should leave the clinic or hospital in the care of a competent adult who can monitor the patient overnight.

Emergency Preparedness

The use of conscious sedation in settings that are remote to the operating room requires that the physician responsible for the conscious sedation be vigilant and prepared for any possible emergent situation. The agents used for conscious sedation may cause loss of protective airway reflexes with inadequate respirations and an obstructed airway. At other times, attempts at conscious sedation fail during a procedure and formal, general anesthesia is needed to successfully complete the procedure. The physician should be prepared for these eventualities.

At a minimum, the physician or dentist should have the appropriate emergency drugs and equipment to address every possible life-threatening complication that may arise from the administration of conscious sedation and should maintain competence in their use. A protocol for the management of emergencies, including calling for specialized assistance, should be developed and emergency drills should be carried out on a regular basis to assess the preparedness of the staff. All of the emergency drugs and equipment should be checked on a regular basis. One should not underestimate the importance of a readily available telephone to summon immediate assistance in an emergency situation.

Written Policies and Procedures

Physicians who administer conscious sedation or supervise the administration of anesthesia for conscious sedation should have written policies and procedures regarding the administration of those anesthetics. The policies and procedures statement should include the minimum qualifications necessary to administer conscious sedation, the standards for evaluating the patient prior to undergoing conscious sedation, the types of monitors that should be used, and standards for documentation of care.

The policies and procedures statement should be prepared by professionals who have extensive experience with the physiology and pharmacology of conscious sedation. This task should not be delegated to administrative personnel who have insufficient understanding of the practice of anesthesiology.

The policies and procedures for conscious sedation should be individualized for the hospital or clinic. Although other hospitals may have common policies and procedures, the temptation to redact policies and procedures verbatim from another hospital should be avoided because the policies and procedures applicable to one institution may not be appropriate for another. Policies copied from another institution may be more detrimental than having no policy at all if the actual practice at the institution conflicts with the stated policy. A defense attorney may be forced into the very difficult position of having to defend both the institution and the professional if the written standards of practice of the institution are at variance with the actual practice of the professional.

Each professional who practices conscious sedation should be responsible for being familiar with the policies and procedures of the institution. These policies and procedures should be periodically monitored and evaluated by the department of anesthesiology and revised on a regular basis to ensure that they continue to reflect actual practice at the institution and that procedures that are outdated or impossible to follow are eliminated.

Responding to Potential Liability

The practitioner should be aware of the federal, state, and hospital requirements for reporting adverse events. When an unexpected adverse event occurs, the appropriate individuals must be informed immediately. It is usually required by law or by hospital bylaws (and is almost always in the practitioner's best interest) to contact the hospital risk management office to report and review the case with the risk manager. Some hospitals convene a medical review committee to investigate an adverse event, especially if the cause of the event is not immediately clear. Many states have passed laws that encourage candid review of these occurrences and, in most instances, internal investigations are protected from the discovery process and subpoena. In states where such laws do not exist, it is important that the parties involved participate in meetings with their attorneys present so that the attorney–client privilege may apply.

Summary

Physicians who wish to administer drugs to achieve conscious sedation in their practices should be familiar with the legal standard of care for the use of conscious sedation and adhere not only to federal regulations and state law but also to the hospital's policy. A sound medical practice based on the legal standard of care will minimize the chance of being held liable for unexpected adverse outcomes.

References

1.   American Dental Association Guidelines for the Use of Conscious Sedation, Deep Sedation and General Anesthesia for Dentists, Adopted by the American Dental Association House of Delegates, October 1999.
2.   American Society of Anesthesiologists (ASA) Position on Monitored Anesthesia Care, December 1998.
3.   Joint Commission on Accreditation of Healthcare Organizations: Comprehensive Accreditation Manual for Hospitals. Chicago, JCAHO, 1997.
4.   Position Statement on the Role of the Registered Nurse (RN) in the Management of Patients Receiving IV Conscious Sedation for Short-Term Therapeutic, Diagnostic, or Surgical Procedures. Endorsed by the American Nurses Association Board of Directors, September 6, 1991.
5.   Practice Guidelines for Sedation and Analgesia by Non-Anesthesiologists: A Report by the American Society of Anesthesiologists Task Force on Sedation and Analgesia by Non-Anesthesiologists. Anesthesiology 84:459–471, 1996.
6.   Projections of Surgical Procedures. Chicago, SMG Marketing Group, Inc., 1999.

Index

Page numbers in **boldface type** indicate complete chapters.